WORKBOOK TO ACCOMPANY

MEDICAL TERMINOLOGY

For Health Professions

7th Edition

Ann Ehrlich
Carol L. Schroeder

D1285796

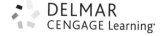

DELMAR
CENGAGE Learning·

Australia • Brazil • Japan • Korea • Mexico • Singapore • Spain • United Kingdom • United States

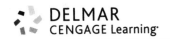

Workbook to Accompany Medical Terminology for Health Professions, Seventh Edition
Ann Ehrlich and Carol L. Schroeder

Vice President, Careers and Computing: Dave Garza

Director of Learning Solutions: Matthew Kane

Senior Acquisitions Editor: Matthew Seeley

Managing Editor: Marah Bellegarde

Senior Product Manager: Debra Myette-Flis

Editorial Assistant: Danielle Yannotti

Vice President, Marketing: Jennifer Baker

Marketing Director: Wendy Mapstone

Senior Marketing Manager: Kristin McNary

Associate Marketing Manager: Jonathan Sheehan

Production Director: Andrew Crouth

Content Project Manager: Thomas Heffernan

Senior Art Director: Jack Pendleton

Technology Project Manager: Patricia Allen

Library of Congress Control Number: 2011945075

ISBN-13: 978-1-111-54328-0

ISBN-10: 1-111-54328-3

Delmar
5 Maxwell Drive
Clifton Park, NY 12065-2919
USA

Cengage Learning products are represented in Canada by Nelson Education, Ltd.

For your lifelong learning solutions, visit **delmar.cengage.com**

Visit our corporate website at **cengage.com**

Notice to the Reader

Printed in the United States of America
2 3 4 5 6 7 16 15 14 13 12

CONTENTS

PREFACE

Our purpose in creating this workbook is to provide you with additional help in mastering the terms and word parts on the **Vocabulary List** shown at the beginning of each chapter. In addition to the learning exercises, there is a crossword puzzle to provide you with a change of pace as you study.

Although the layout of the workbook is similar to the learning exercises in your textbook, these are all new questions. You have not seen them before, and these exercises place more emphasis on the use of word parts in learning medical terminology.

The answer keys for these questions **are not** in the workbook. Your instructor will explain how these exercises are to be corrected and graded. Answers to the crossword puzzles are at the back of the workbook; however, unless you have been told otherwise, this is an optional, not for credit, activity.

We suggest that the exercises be graded on a pass-fail basis. Don't be fooled by this seemingly simple system. Your individual score is important because it provides feedback as to how well you are doing with your studies.

- A score of 70 to 75 is passing and excellent. Congratulations!

- A score of 65 to 69 is still passing; however, it indicates that you need more work toward your mastery of these terms.

- A score of 64 or lower is failing and shows that you need to study more! The time to seek help is now—before you fall behind on the chapters that follow.

We wish you well with your study of medical terminology and in your healthcare career.

Ann Ehrlich
Carol L. Schroeder

Introduction to Medical Terminology

Learning Exercises

Class _____ Name _____

Matching Word Parts #1

Write the correct answer in the middle column.

Definition	Correct Answer	Possible Answers
1.1. abnormal condition	_____	-algia
1.2. deficient	_____	-ectomy
1.3. excessive	_____	hyper-
1.4. pain	_____	hypo-
1.5. surgical removal	_____	-osis

Matching Word Parts #2

Write the correct answer in the middle column.

Definition	Correct Answer	Possible Answers
1.6. bursting forth of blood	_____	-plasty
1.7. flow or discharge	_____	-rrhage
1.8. rupture	_____	-rrhaphy
1.9. surgical repair	_____	-rrhea
1.10. surgical suturing	_____	-rrhexis

Matching Word Parts #3

Write the correct answer in the middle column.

Definition	Correct Answer	Possible Answers
1.11. abnormal hardening	_____	-sclerosis
1.12. a surgical incision	_____	-otomy
1.13. bad, difficult, painful	_____	-ostomy
1.14. an artificial opening	_____	-itis
1.15. inflammation	_____	dys-

Fill in the Blank #1

1.16. A/An _____ is the invasion of the body by a disease-producing organism.

1.17. A/An _____ is a word, such as *laser*, which is formed from the initial letter, or letters, of the major parts of a compound term.

1.18. The term _____ means between, but not within, the parts of a tissue.

1.19. The term _____ describes swelling caused by an abnormal accumulation of fluid in the body tissues.

1.20. The term _____ describes a disease named for the person who first discovered it.

Word Construction #1

Use these word parts to construct the term that answers the following questions. Combining vowels are used in the term only when necessary. The answer includes the term (plus the appropriate word parts). For example: *hepatitis* (hepat, -itis).

-al	-algia	angi/o	enter/o	gastr/o	-graphy	hem/o	hepat/o
-itis	-megaly	nat/o	neo-	-ology	-osis	path/o	-rrhage

1.21. The process of producing a radiographic study of the blood vessels is known as _____.

1.22. Enlargement of the liver is described by the term _____.

1.23. The term _____ means pain in the stomach.

1.24. A/An _____ is the loss of a large amount of blood in a short time.

1.25. The study of all aspects of diseases is known as _____.

1.26. The term _____ describes the study of disorders of the newborn.

1.27. An inflammation of the stomach is known as _____.

1.28. The term _____ describes an inflammation of the stomach and small intestine.

1.29. The term _____ means pertaining to birth.

1.30. The term _____ means any disease of the stomach.

Matching Medical Terms and Definitions #1

Write the correct answer in the middle column.

Definitions	Correct Answer	Possible Answers
1.31. abnormal passage between organs	_____	diagnosis
1.32. cracklike sore of the skin	_____	fissure
1.33. identification of a disease	_____	fistula
1.34. general discomfort	_____	malaise
1.35. prediction of disease outcome	_____	prognosis

Word Surgery #1

Divide these terms into word parts, in the proper sequence, on the lines provided to create the answer to the question. Use a slash (/) to indicate a combining form. Use a hyphen to indicate a prefix or suffix. (You may not need all of the lines provided.)

1.36. An **appendectomy** is the surgical removal of the appendix.

_____   _____   _____   _____

1.37. The term **arthralgia** means pain in a joint or joints.

_____   _____   _____   _____

1.38. A **colostomy** is the surgical creation of an artificial excretory opening between the colon and the body surface.

_____   _____   _____   _____

1.39. **Otorhinolaryngology** is the study of the ears, nose, and throat.

_____   _____   _____   _____

1.40. A **dermatologist** is a physician who specializes in diagnosing and treating disorders of the skin.

_____   _____   _____   _____

Fill in the Blank #2

1.41. A/An _____ is a localized response to an injury or destruction of tissues.

1.42. Pain is classified as a/an _____.

1.43. The medical screening of patients to determine their relative priority of need and the proper place of treatment is known as _____.

1.44. A/An _____ is a torn or jagged wound or an accidental cut wound.

1.45. A/An _____ is a set of the signs and symptoms that occur together.

Multiple Choice

Select the correct answer and write it on the line provided.

1.46. The act of rotating the arm so that the palm of the hand is forward or upward is known as _____.

    supination   suppuration

1.47. A _____ is a pathologic change of the tissues due to disease or injury.

    laceration   lesion

1.48. The term _____ describes an examination technique in which the examiner's hands are used to feel the texture, size, consistency, and location of certain body parts.

    palpation   palpitation

1.49. The term _____ describes higher than normal blood pressure.

    hypertension   hypotension

1.50. The term _____ describes any pathologic change or disease in the spinal cord.

    myelopathy   myopathy

Word Construction #2

Use these word parts to construct the term that answers the following questions. Combining vowels are used in the term only when necessary. The answer includes the term (plus the appropriate word parts). For example: *hepatitis* (hepat, -itis).

-al	arteri/o	end-	-itis	my/o	myc/o	myel	neur/o
-osis	-pathy	poli/o	pyr/o	-rrhaphy	-rrhexis	-sclerosis	tonsill/o

1.51. The term _____ describes any abnormal condition or disease caused by a fungus.

1.52. The term _____ describes any pathologic change or disease of muscle tissue.

1.53. Discomfort due to the regurgitation of stomach acid upward into the esophagus is known as _____.

1.54. The term _____ describes suturing together the ends of a severed nerve.

1.55. A viral infection of the gray matter of the spinal cord is known as _____.

1.56. The term _____ means pertaining to the interior or lining of an artery.

1.57. The rupture of a muscle is known as _____.

1.58. The term _____ describes the abnormal hardening of the walls of an artery or arteries.

1.59. The _____ means inflammation of the tonsils.

Matching Medical Terms and Definitions #2

Write the correct answer in the middle column.

Definitions	Correct Answer	Possible Answers
1.60. above the ribs	_____	acute
1.61. objective evidence of disease	_____	palpitation
1.62. pertaining to a virus	_____	sign
1.63. pounding, racing heart	_____	supracostal
1.64. rapid onset	_____	trauma
1.65. wound or injury	_____	viral

Word Surgery #2

Divide these terms into word parts, in the proper sequence, on the lines provided to create the answer to the question. Use a slash (/) to indicate a combining form. Use a hyphen to indicate a prefix or suffix. (You may not need all of the lines provided.)

1.66. **Abdominocentesis** is the surgical puncture of the abdominal cavity to remove fluid.

_____ _____ _____ _____

1.67. **Diarrhea** is the flow of frequent loose or watery stools.

_____ _____ _____ _____

1.68. An **erythrocyte** is a mature red blood cell.

_____ _____ _____ _____

1.69. The term **cyanosis** describes blue discoloration of the skin caused by a lack of adequate oxygen in the blood.

_____ _____ _____ _____

1.70. The term **pyoderma** describes any acute, inflammatory, pus-forming bacterial skin infection such as impetigo.

_____ _____ _____ _____

Fill in the Blank #3

1.71. The term _____ describes the formation or discharge of pus.

1.72. Lower than normal blood pressure is known as _____.

1.73. The term _____ means within the muscle.

1.74. The _____ are the bones of the fingers and toes.

1.75. A/An _____ is the temporary, partial, or complete disappearance of the symptoms.

CHAPTER 1 CROSSWORD PUZZLE

The answers for this puzzle are located at the back of this workbook on page 93.

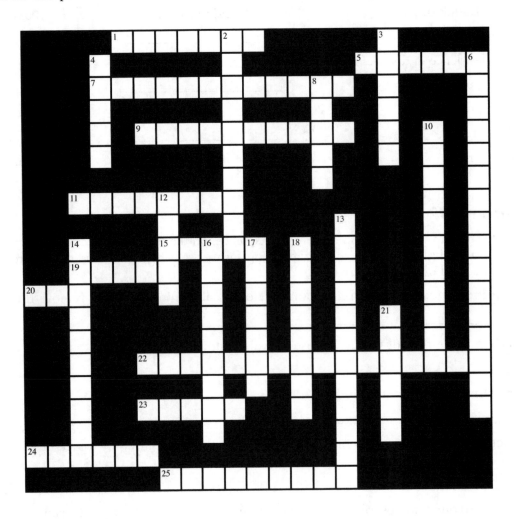

ACROSS

1. Suffix meaning surgical suturing
5. Wound or injury
7. A localized response to injury or destruction of tissues
9. Torn, ragged wound
11. The frequent flow of loose or watery stools
15. Prefix meaning excessive or increased
19. Rapid onset of disease and a relatively short duration
20. Prefix meaning bad, difficult, or painful
22. A surgical puncture into the abdomen to remove fluid
23. Suffix meaning pain and suffering
24. Suffix meaning surgical repair
25. Surgical creation of an artificial excretory opening between the colon and the body surface

DOWN

2. The loss of a large amount of blood in a short time
3. Medical screening to determine the priority of treatment
4. Pertaining to a virus
6. Abnormal hardening of the walls of an artery or arteries
8. Suffix meaning a surgical incision
10. Inflammation of the tonsils
12. Suffix meaning flow or discharge
13. Surgical removal of the appendix
14. Pain in the stomach
16. Prediction of probable course and outcome of a disorder
17. Suffix meaning rupture
18. A set of signs and symptoms that occur together
21. Suffix meaning surgical creation of an artificial opening to the body surface

The Human Body in Health and Disease

Learning Exercises

Class _____   Name _____

Matching Word Parts #1

Write the correct answer in the middle column.

Definition	Correct Answer	Possible Answers
2.1. cell	_____	-ologist
2.2. fat	_____	hist/o
2.3. gland	_____	cyt/o
2.4. specialist	_____	adip/o
2.5. tissue	_____	aden/o

Matching Word Parts #2

Write the correct answer in the middle column.

Definition	Correct Answer	Possible Answers
2.6. back	_____	anter/o
2.7. control	_____	caud/o
2.8. front	_____	cephal/o
2.9. head	_____	poster/o
2.10. lower part of body	_____	-stasis

Matching Word Parts #3

Write the correct answer in the middle column.

Definition	Correct Answer	Possible Answers
2.11. disease, suffering, emotion	_____	endo-
2.12. out of	_____	exo-
2.13. formation	_____	-ology
2.14. study of	_____	path/o
2.15. within	_____	-plasia

Fill in the Blank #1

2.16. A/An _____ is a horizontal plane that divides the body into upper and lower portions.

2.17. An unfavorable response due to prescribed medical treatment is known as a/an _____ illness.

2.18. The _____ is the space formed by the hip bones that primarily contains the organs of the reproductive and excretory systems.

2.19. A/An _____ is a pathologic condition caused by an absent or defective gene.

2.20. Unspecialized cells that renew themselves for long periods of time through cell division are known as _____.

Word Construction #1

Use these word parts to construct the term that answers the following questions. Combining vowels are used in the term only when necessary. The answer includes the term (plus the appropriate word parts). For example: *hepatitis* (hepat, -itis).

aden/o	ana-	carcin/o	dys-	-ectomy	endo-	hyper-	hypo-
-ia	-malacia	-oma	-osis	-plasia	-sclerosis	-stenosis	-trophy

2.21. The term _____ describes the abnormal softening of a gland.

2.22. The term _____ describes a change in the structure of cells and in their orientation to each other.

2.23. The abnormal hardening of a gland is known as _____.

2.24. The term _____ describes the enlargement of an organ or tissue because of an abnormal increase in the number of cells in the tissues.

2.25. A/An _____ is a benign tumor that arises in or resembles glandular tissue.

2.26. The term _____ describes a general increase in the bulk of a body part due to an increase in the size, but not in the number, of cells in the tissues.

2.27. The surgical procedure to remove a gland is known as a/an _____.

2.28. The incomplete development of an organ or tissue, usually due to a deficiency in the number of cells, is known as _____.

2.29. The abnormal development or growth of cells, tissues, or organs is known as _____.

2.30. A/An _____ is a malignant tumor that originates in glandular tissue.

Matching Medical Terms and Definitions #1

Write the correct answer in the middle column.

Definitions	Correct Answer	Possible Answers
2.31. belly button or navel	_____	anomaly
2.32. deviation from normal	_____	geriatrician
2.33. relating to the groin	_____	inguinal
2.34. situated nearest the midline	_____	proximal
2.35. specialist caring for older people	_____	umbilicus

Word Surgery

Divide these terms into word parts, in the proper sequence, on the lines provided to create the answer to the question. Use a slash (/) to indicate a combining form. Use a hyphen to indicate a prefix or suffix. (You may not need all of the lines provided.)

2.36. The **hypogastric** region is located below the stomach.

_____ _____ _____ _____

2.37. The term **caudal** means toward the lower part of the body.

_____ _____ _____ _____

2.38. **Aplasia** is the defective development or the congenital absence of an organ or tissue.

_____ _____ _____ _____

2.39. The term **cephalic** means toward the head.

_____ _____ _____ _____

2.40. **Physiology** is the study of the functions of the structures of the body.

_____ _____ _____ _____

Fill in the Blank #2

2.41. The term _____ means situated in the back. It also means on the back part of an organ.

2.42. The genetic structures located within the nucleus of each cell are known as _____.

2.43. The group of hereditary bleeding disorders in which a blood-clotting factor is missing is known as _____.

2.44. A/An _____ disorder is an illness without known cause.

2.45. The _____ contains primarily the major organs of digestion.

Multiple Choice

Select the correct answer and write it on the line provided.

2.46. The term _____ means situated in the front. It also means on the front or forward part of an organ.

    anterior   posterior

2.47. The condition known as _____ is a genetic disorder in which the essential digestive enzyme phenylalanine hydroxylase is missing.

    phenylketonuria   Tay-Sachs disease

2.48. The spread of a disease by the bite of a certain mosquito is known as _____ transmission.

    bloodborne   vector-borne

2.49. An _____ gland secretes one or more hormones directly into the bloodstream.

    endocrine   exocrine

2.50. A _____ disorder produces symptoms for which no physiological or anatomical cause can be identified.

    congenital   functional

Word Construction #2

Use these word parts to construct the term that answers the following questions. Combining vowels are used in the term only when necessary. The answer includes the term (plus the appropriate word parts). For example: *hepatitis* (hepat, -itis).

-al	-crine	cyt/o	dem/o	-eal	en-	endo-
epi-	eti-	exo-	hist/o	home/o	-ic	-itis
-ology	-osis	pan-	periton/o	-plasm	retro-	-stasis

2.51. The term _____ means located behind the peritoneum.

2.52. The term _____ means the study of the causes of diseases.

2.53. The material within the cell membrane that is *not* part of the nucleus is known as _____.

2.54. The _____ glands secrete chemical substances into ducts that lead either to other organs or out of the body.

2.55. A/An _____ is a sudden and widespread outbreak of a disease within a specific population group or area.

2.56. The study of the structure, composition, and function of tissues is known as _____.

2.57. The term _____ describes an inflammation of the peritoneum.

2.58. The ongoing presence of a disease within a population, group, or area is known as being _____.

2.59. The processes through which the body maintains a constant internal environment is known as _____.

2.60. A/An _____ is an outbreak of a disease occurring over a large geographic area, possibly worldwide.

Matching Medical Terms and Definitions #2

Write the correct answer in the middle column.

Definitions	Correct Answer	Possible Answers
2.61. back of the body and head	_____	anatomy
2.62. farthest from the midline	_____	distal
2.63. front (belly side) of the body	_____	dorsal
2.64. region above the stomach	_____	epigastric
2.65. study of the structures of the body	_____	medial
2.66. toward the midline	_____	ventral

Fill in the Blank #3

2.67. A/An _____ is any condition that is transmitted from one person to another by either direct or indirect contact with contaminated objects.

2.68. The spread of a disease through contact with blood or other body fluids that have been contaminated with blood is known as _____.

2.69. The _____ is a fused double layer of the parietal peritoneum that attaches parts of the intestine to the interior abdominal wall.

2.70. The _____ divides the body into equal left and right halves.

2.71. A/An _____ is an illness caused by living pathogenic organisms such as bacteria and viruses.

2.72. The multilayered membrane that protects and holds the organs in place within the abdominal cavity is known as the _____.

2.73. A/An _____ is an abnormal condition that exists at the time of birth.

2.74. The _____ surrounds and protects the heart and the lungs.

2.75. A disease acquired in a hospital or clinic setting is known as a/an _____.

CHAPTER 2 CROSSWORD PUZZLE

The answers for this puzzle are located at the back of this workbook on page 94.

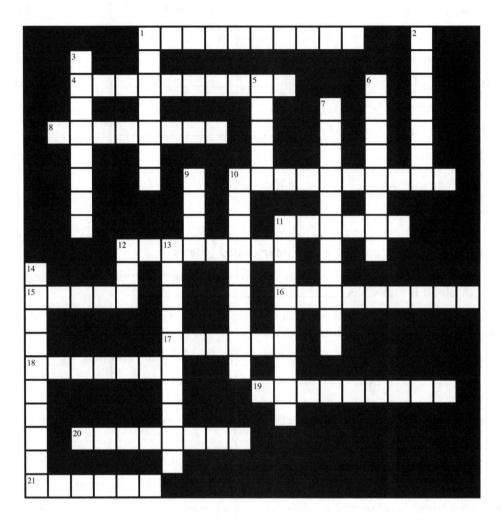

ACROSS

1. Surgical removal of a gland
4. An infection acquired in a hospital or clinic
8. Term meaning toward the head
10. Abnormal condition that exists at the time of birth
11. Situated farthest from the midline
12. Study of the causes of diseases
15. Combining form meaning disease
16. Situated in back
17. Suffix meaning formation
18. Defective development or congenital absence of an organ or tissue
19. The study of tissues
20. Situated nearest the midline
21. Toward the lower part of the body

DOWN

1. A deviation from normal
2. A benign tumor of glandular origin
3. Situated in the front
5. Combining form meaning fat
6. Term meaning relating to the groin
7. Maintaining a constant internal environment
9. Prefix meaning within
10. Material within the cell membrane that is not part of the nucleus
11. Abnormal growth of cells, tissue, or organs
12. Prefix meaning out of
13. Disorder without known cause
14. Region located above the stomach

The Skeletal System

Learning Exercises

Class _____   Name _____

Matching Word Parts #1

Write the correct answer in the middle column.

Definition	Correct Answer	Possible Answers
3.1. curve, swayback bent	_____	chondr/o
3.2. bone marrow, spinal cord	_____	crani/o
3.3. bone	_____	lord/o
3.4. cartilage	_____	myel/o
3.5. cranium	_____	oss/i, oste/o, ost/o

Matching Word Parts #2

Write the correct answer in the middle column.

Definition	Correct Answer	Possible Answers
3.6. crooked, bent, or stiff	_____	ankyl/o
3.7. curved	_____	arthr/o
3.8. hump	_____	kyph/o
3.9. joint	_____	scoli/o
3.10. singular noun ending	_____	-um

Matching Word Parts #3

Write the correct answer in the middle column.

Definition	Correct Answer	Possible Answers
3.11. to bind, tie together	_____	synovi/o, synov/o
3.12. rib	_____	spondyl/o
3.13. setting free, loosening	_____	-lysis
3.14. synovial membrane	_____	-desis
3.15. vertebra, vertebrae	_____	cost/o

Fill in the Blank #1

3.16. The condition known as _____ is a chronic autoimmune disorder in which the joints and some organs of other body systems are attacked.

3.17. _____ is a bone disease characterized by the excessive breakdown of bone tissue that is followed by abnormal bone formation.

3.18. Dual x-ray _____ is a low-exposure radiographic measurement of the spine and hips to evaluate bone density.

3.19. A/An _____ is a mechanical appliance such as a leg brace or splint that is specially designed to control, correct, or compensate for impaired limb function.

3.20. A/An _____ hip fracture is usually caused by weakening of the bones due to osteoporosis. It can occur either spontaneously or as the result of a fall.

Word Construction #1

Use these word parts to construct the term that answers the following questions. Combining vowels are used in the term only when necessary. The answer includes the term (plus the appropriate word parts). For example: *hepatitis* (hepat, -itis).

arthr/o	chondr/o	-clasis	-desis	-itis	-malacia	myel/o	-necrosis
-oma	-osis	ost/o	oste/o	-penia	por/o	-rrhaphy	-rrhexis

3.21. The surgical fracture of a bone to correct a deformity is known as _____.

3.22. The term _____ describes thinner than average bone density.

3.23. The death of bone tissue due to a lack of insufficient blood supply is known as _____.

3.24. The term _____ describes the surgical suturing, or wiring together, of bones.

3.25. A/An _____ is a benign bony projection covered with cartilage.

3.26. The term _____ refers to a marked loss of bone density and an increase in bone porosity commonly associated with aging.

3.27. An inflammation of bone is known as _____.

3.28. The term _____ describes abnormal softening of bones in adults.

3.29. An inflammation of the bone marrow and adjacent bone is known as _____.

3.30. The condition of _____ is commonly known as wear-and-tear arthritis.

Matching Fractures and Definitions

Write the correct answer in the middle column.

Definitions	Correct Answer	Type of Fracture
3.31. bone splintered or crushed	_____	comminuted
3.32. bone pieces pressed together	_____	compression
3.33. bone twisted apart	_____	open
3.34. break of weakened bone	_____	pathologic
3.35. break with an open wound	_____	spiral

Word Surgery

Divide these terms into word parts, in the proper sequence, on the lines provided to create the answer to the question. Use a slash (/) to indicate a combining form. Use a hyphen to indicate a prefix or suffix. (You may not need all of the lines provided.)

3.36. A **podiatrist** specializes in diagnosing and treating disorders of the feet.

_____   _____   _____   _____

3.37. **Arthrodesis** is the surgical fusion of two bones to stiffen a joint.

_____   _____   _____   _____

3.38. **Craniostenosis** is a malformation of the skull due to the premature closure of the cranial sutures.

_____   _____   _____   _____

3.39. **Costochondritis** is an inflammation of the cartilage that connects a rib to the sternum.

_____   _____   _____   _____

3.40. **Hemopoietic** means pertaining to the formation of blood cells.

_____   _____   _____   _____

Fill in the Blank #2

3.41. A/An _____ is an artificial substitute for a diseased or missing body part such as a leg that has been amputated.

3.42. The condition in children that is characterized by defective bone growth is known as _____.

3.43. A/An _____ is a physician who specializes in diagnosing and treating diseases and disorders involving the bones, joints, and muscles.

3.44. The grating sound heard when the ends of a broken bone move together is known as _____.

3.45. The visual examination of the internal structure of a joint is known as _____.

Multiple Choice

Select the correct answer and write it on the line provided.

3.46. The term _____ describes the surgical loosening of an ankylosed joint.

  arthrodesis   arthrolysis

3.47. The term _____ means originating within an individual.

  allogenic   autologous

3.48. A/An _____ is an abnormal enlargement of the joint at the base of the great toe.

  fibrous dysplasia   hallux valgus

3.49. The _____ are the five bones that form the palms of the hand.

  metacarpals   metatarsals

3.50. A fracture treatment in which a plate or pins are placed directly into the bone to hold the broken pieces in place is known as _____.

  external fixation   internal fixation

Word Construction #2

Use these word parts to construct the term that answers the following questions. Combining vowels are used in the term only when necessary. The answer includes the term (plus the appropriate word parts). For example: *hepatitis* (hepat, -itis).

arthr/o	chondr/o	-ectomy	hem/o	-itis	lamin/o	-listhesis	-malacia
myel/o	-oma	-osis	ost/o	peri-	scoli/o	spondyl/o	synov/o

3.51. The term _____ describes an abnormal lateral curvature of the spine.

3.52. A/An _____ is a slow-growing benign tumor derived from cartilage cells.

3.53. The forward movement of the body of one of the lower lumbar vertebra on the vertebra below it is known as _____.

3.54. The abnormal softening of cartilage is known as _____.

3.55. The degenerative disorder that can cause the loss of normal spinal structure and function is known as _____.

3.56. A/An _____ is a type of cancer that occurs in blood-making cells found in the red bone marrow.

3.57. The term _____ is an inflammation of the periosteum.

3.58. The surgical removal of a lamina, or posterior portion, of a vertebra is known as a/an _____.

3.59. Blood within a joint is known as _____.

3.60. A/An _____ is the surgical removal of a synovial membrane from a joint.

Matching Medical Terms and Definitions

Write the correct answer in the middle column.

Definitions	Correct Answer	Possible Answers
3.61. ankle bony protuberance	_____	acetabulum
3.62. hip socket	_____	malleolus
3.63. segments of the spinal column	_____	manubrium
3.64. upper portion of sternum	_____	metatarsals
3.65. where toes attach to the foot	_____	vertebrae

Fill in the Blank #3

3.66. An abnormal increase in the forward curvature of the lumbar spine is known as _____.

3.67. The condition known as _____ is a congenital defect of the spine that develops during early pregnancy.

3.68. The partial displacement of a bone from its joint is known as _____.

3.69. The term _____ means originating within another.

3.70. The form of rheumatoid arthritis characterized by progressive stiffening of the spine is known as _____.

3.71. The term _____ is a bone disorder of unknown cause that destroys normal bone structure and replaces it with scarlike tissue.

3.72. Juvenile _____ is an autoimmune disorder that affects children of 16 years of age or less with symptoms that include stiffness, pain, joint swelling, skin rash, fever, slowed growth, and fatigue.

3.73. A/An _____ is performed to treat osteoporosis-related compression fractures.

3.74. The term _____ describes pain of the lumbar region of the spine.

3.75. The condition known as _____ is an abnormal increase in the outward curvature of the thoracic spine as viewed from the side.

CHAPTER 3 CROSSWORD PUZZLE

The answers for this puzzle are located at the back of this workbook on page 95.

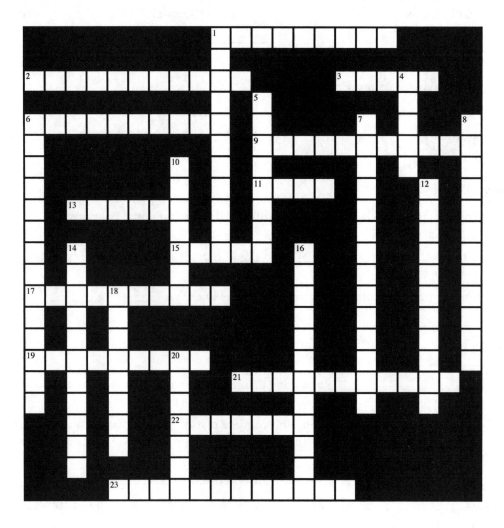

ACROSS

1. An abnormal lateral curvature of the spine
2. The partial displacement of a bone from its joint
3. Combining form meaning bone marrow
6. A fracture in which the bone is splintered or crushed
9. Inflammation of the periosteum
11. A fracture in which there is an open wound in the skin
13. Combining form meaning crooked, bent, or stiff
15. Suffix meaning to bind, tie together
17. Originating within an individual
19. Benign tumor of cartilage cells
21. Pertaining to blood cell formation
22. Low back pain
23. Blood within a joint space

DOWN

1. Degenerative condition that can cause the loss of normal spinal structure
4. Suffix meaning loosening or setting free
5. Humpback
6. Abnormal softening of the cartilage
7. Form of arthritis commonly associated with aging
8. Abnormal softening of bones due to disease
10. Combining form meaning cartilage
12. Surgical loosening of an ankylosed joint
14. Visual examination of the internal structure of a joint
16. Marked loss of bone density frequently associated with aging
18. Swayback
20. A type of cancer that occurs in the red bone marrow

The Muscular System

Learning Exercises

Class _____ Name _____

Matching Word Parts #1

Write the correct answer in the middle column.

Definition	Correct Answer	Possible Answers
4.1. bad	_____	bi-
4.2. hernia	_____	-cele
4.3. muscle	_____	dys-
4.4. paralysis	_____	my/o
4.5. two	_____	-plegia

Matching Word Parts #2

Write the correct answer in the middle column.

Definition	Correct Answer	Possible Answers
4.6. abnormal condition	_____	fasci/o
4.7. fascia	_____	fibr/o
4.8. fibrous tissue	_____	-ia
4.9. movement	_____	kinesi/o
4.10. three	_____	tri-

Matching Word Parts #3

Write the correct answer in the middle column.

Definition	Correct Answer	Possible Answers
4.11. coordination	_____	ton/o
4.12. pertaining to	_____	ten/o, tend/o
4.13. rupture	_____	tax/o
4.14. tendon	_____	-rrhexis
4.15. tone	_____	-ic

Fill in the Blank #1

4.16. The term _____ means slanted or at an angle.

4.17. Jerking of the limbs that can occur normally as a person is falling asleep is known as _____.

4.18. The condition known as _____ occurs when inflamed and swollen tendons are caught in the narrow space between the bones within the shoulder joint.

4.19. A/An _____ is a specialist who works under a physician's supervision to develop, implement, and coordinate exercise programs, and administer medical tests to promote physical fitness.

4.20. A calcium deposit in the plantar fascia near its attachment to the calcaneus (heel) bone is known as a/an _____.

Word Construction #1

Use these word parts to construct the term that answers the following questions. Combining vowels are used in the term only when necessary. The answer includes the term (plus the appropriate word parts). For example: *hepatitis* (hepat, -itis).

-cele	clon/o	hemi-	hyper-	hypo-	-ia	-itis	kines/o	-lysis
my/o	myos/o	-para	-paresis	poly-	-rrhaphy	ton/o	-us	

4.21. The term _____ describes the sudden, involuntary jerking of a muscle or group of muscles.

4.22. The muscle disease characterized by the inflammation and weakening of voluntary muscles in many parts of the body at the same time is known as _____.

4.23. The term _____ describes abnormally increased muscle function or activity.

4.24. The condition in which there is diminished tone of the skeletal muscles is known as _____.

4.25. A/An _____ is the protrusion of muscle substance through a tear in the surrounding fascia.

4.26. The term _____ describes a weakness or slight muscular paralysis.

4.27. The degeneration of muscle tissue is known as _____.

4.28. The term _____ means slight paralysis or weakness in one side of the body.

4.29. The surgical suturing a muscle wound is known as _____.

4.30. The term _____ describes the loss of sensation and voluntary muscle movements.

Matching Movements and Definitions

Write the correct answer in the middle column.

Definitions	Correct Answer	Movement
4.31. bends the foot upward at the ankle	_____	abduction
4.32. circular movement at the far end of a limb	_____	adduction
4.33. moves away from the midline	_____	circumduction
4.34. moves toward the midline	_____	dorsiflexion
4.35. turns the palm of the hand downward or backward	_____	pronation

Word Surgery

Divide these terms into word parts, in the proper sequence, on the lines provided to create the answer to the question. Use a slash (/) to indicate a combining form. Use a hyphen to indicate a prefix or suffix. (You may not need all of the lines provided.)

4.36. **Tenosynovitis** is an inflammation of the sheath surrounding a tendon.

_____   _____   _____   _____

4.37. **Fibromyalgia** syndrome is a debilitating chronic condition characterized by fatigue, diffuse and/or specific muscle, joint, or bone pain, and a wide range of other symptoms.

_____   _____   _____   _____

4.38. **Epicondylitis** is inflammation of the tissues surrounding the elbow.

_____   _____   _____   _____

4.39. **Myofascial** release is a specialized soft-tissue manipulation technique used to ease the pain of conditions such as fibromyalgia.

_____   _____   _____   _____

4.40. Plantar **fasciitis** is an inflammation of the plantar fascia on the sole of the foot.

_____   _____   _____   _____

Fill in the Blank #2

4.41. A/An _____ specializes in physical medicine and rehabilitation with the focus on restoring function.

4.42. The painful condition caused by the muscle tearing away from the tibia is known as a/an _____.

4.43. Chronic _____ (CFS) is characterized by profound fatigue that is not improved by bed rest and may be made worse by physical or mental activity.

4.44. The general term _____ describes a group of genetic diseases characterized by progressive weakness and degeneration of the skeletal muscles without affecting the nervous system.

4.45. The term _____ describes a stiff neck due to a contraction of the neck muscles that pull the head toward the affected side.

Multiple Choice

Select the correct answer and write it on the line provided.

4.46. A/An _____ is a ringlike muscle that tightly constricts the opening of a passageway.

    singultus   sphincter

4.47. An injury to a joint, such as the ankle, knee, or wrist, that usually involves a wrenched or torn ligament is known as a _____.

    sprain   strain

4.48. The term _____ describes slight paralysis or weakness affecting one side of the body.

    hemiparesis   hemiplegia

4.49. The term _____ describes pain in the leg muscles that occurs during exercise and is relieved by rest.

    intermittent claudication   myasthenia gravis

4.50. A harmless fluid-filled swelling that occurs most commonly on the outer surface of the wrist is known as a _____.

    carpal tunnel   ganglion cyst

Word Construction #2

Use these word parts to construct the term that answers the following questions. Combining vowels are used in the term only when necessary. The answer includes the term (plus the appropriate word parts). For example: *hepatitis* (hepat, -itis).

a-	brady-	-desis	-dynia	dys-	-ia	-ic	kines/o
-lysis	-rrhaphy	-rrhexis	tax/o	ten/o	ton/o	-trophy	

4.51. The term _____ is surgical suturing together of the divided ends of a tendon.

4.52. Weakness or wearing away of body tissues and structures is known as _____.

4.53. The term _____ describes the inability to coordinate muscle activity during voluntary movement.

4.54. The surgical suturing of the end of a tendon to bone is known as _____.

4.55. The term _____ describes a condition of abnormal muscle tone that causes the impairment of voluntary muscle movement.

4.56. The term _____ means lacking normal muscle tone or strength.

4.57. The term _____ means extreme slowness in movement.

4.58. The distortion or impairment of voluntary movement, such as a tic or spasm, is known as _____.

4.59. The release of a tendon from adhesions is known as _____.

4.60. The term muscular _____ refers to a group of genetic diseases characterized by progressive weakness.

Matching Medical Terms and Definitions

Write the correct answer in the middle column.

Definitions	Correct Answer	Possible Answers
4.61. elastic connective tissues are replaced with nonelastic fibrous tissues	_____	contracture
4.62. loss of sensation and voluntary movements in a muscle	_____	hemiplegia
4.63. paralysis of all four extremities	_____	paralysis
4.64. paralysis of entire lower part of the body	_____	paraplegia
4.65. total paralysis of one side of the body	_____	quadriplegia

Fill in the Blank #3

4.66. A/An _____ is a band of fibrous tissue that holds structures together abnormally.

4.67. Myoclonus of the diaphragm that causes the characteristic hiccup sound with each spasm is known as _____.

4.68. The symptoms of _____ syndrome occur when the tendons that pass through the carpal tunnel are chronically overused and become inflamed and swollen.

4.69. The diagnostic test that measures the electrical activity within muscle fibers in response to nerve stimulation is known as _____.

4.70. The term _____ describes the study of the human factors that affect the design and operation of tools and the work environment.

4.71. The term _____ describes the chronic autoimmune disease that affects the neuro-muscular junction and produces serious weakness of voluntary muscles.

4.72. The loss of muscle mass, strength, and function that comes with aging is known as _____.

4.73. The term _____ describes weakness or wearing away of body tissues and structures.

4.74. Inflammation of a fascia is known as _____.

4.75. The term _____ describes abnormally increased muscle function or activity.

CHAPTER 4 CROSSWORD PUZZLE

The answers for this puzzle are located at the back of this workbook on page 96.

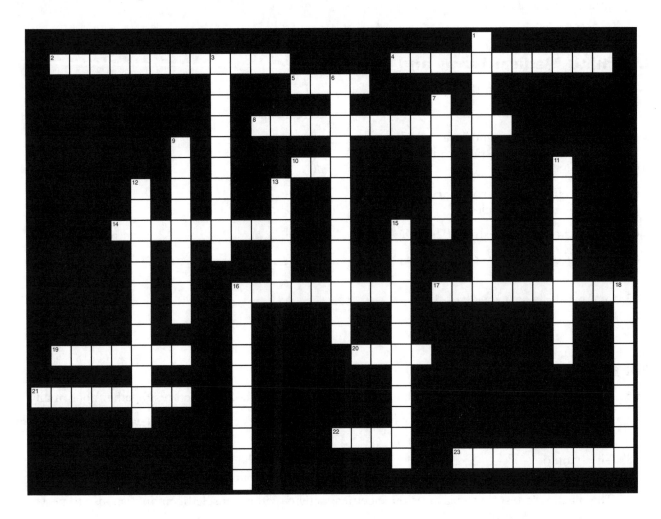

ACROSS

2. Extreme slowness in movement
4. A slight paralysis affecting one side of the body
5. Combining form meaning tone
8. Circular movement at the far end of a limb
10. Combining form meaning muscle
14. Ring-like muscle
16. Hiccups
17. The distortion or impairment of voluntary movement such as a tic
19. Hernia of a muscle through the fascia surrounding it
20. Suffix meaning hernia
21. A band of fibrous tissue that holds structures together abnormally
22. Combining form meaning coordination
23. Movement toward the midline

DOWN

1. Inflammation of tissues surrounding the elbow
3. The study of human factors that affect tools and the work environment
6. Relationship between a nerve and muscle
7. Weakness and wearing away of tissue and structures
9. Inflammation of fascia
11. Paralysis of the lower part of the body
12. Abnormally increased muscle function or activity
13. A stretched or torn ligament in a joint
15. Bending the foot upward at the ankle
16. Age-related loss of muscle mass
18. Movement away from the midline

The Cardiovascular System

Learning Exercises

Class _____   Name _____

Matching Word Parts #1

Write the correct answer in the middle column.

Definition	Correct Answer	Possible Answers
5.1. aorta	_____	angi/o
5.2. artery	_____	aort/o
5.3. mixture or blending	_____	arteri/o
5.4. vein	_____	-crasia
5.5. vessel	_____	phleb/o

Matching Word Parts #2

Write the correct answer in the middle column.

Definition	Correct Answer	Possible Answers
5.6. plaque or fatty substance	_____	ven/o
5.7. red	_____	leuk/o
5.8. slow	_____	erythr/o
5.9. vein	_____	brady-
5.10. white	_____	ather/o

Matching Word Parts #3

Write the correct answer in the middle column.

Definition	Correct Answer	Possible Answers
5.11. blood condition	_____	card/o, cardi/o
5.12. blood	_____	-emia
5.13. clot	_____	hem/o, hemat/o
5.14. heart	_____	tachy-
5.15. fast	_____	thromb/o

Fill in the Blank #1

5.16. Low blood pressure that occurs upon standing up is known as _____.

5.17. An automated _____ (AED) is designed for use by nonprofessionals in emergency situations when defibrillation is required.

5.18. The group of bone marrow disorders characterized by the insufficient production of one or more types of blood cells due to dysfunction of the bone marrow is known as _____ syndrome.

5.19. A/An _____ is a serious complication of a blood transfusion in which a severe immune response occurs because the patient's blood and the donated blood do not match.

5.20. A/An _____ blocks the action of the enzyme that causes the blood vessels to contract, resulting in hypertension.

Word Construction #1

Use these word parts to construct the term that answers the following questions. Combining vowels are used in the term only when necessary. The answer includes the term (plus the appropriate word parts). For example: *hepatitis* (hepat, -itis).

ather/o	-cytes	-ectomy	embol/o	-emia	-ism	-itis
leuk/o	-oma	-osis	-penia	-sclerosis	thromb/o	-us

5.21. The term _____ describes a type of cancer characterized by a progressive increase in the number of abnormal white blood cells found in blood-forming tissues.

5.22. The surgical removal of plaque buildup from the interior of an artery is known as a/an _____.

5.23. A/An _____ is a blood clot attached to the interior wall of an artery or vein.

5.24. The sudden blockage of a blood vessel by an embolus is known as a/an _____.

5.25. A/An _____ is a deposit of plaque on or within the arterial wall.

5.26. The term _____ describes any situation in which the total number of leukocytes in the circulating blood is less than normal.

5.27. A/An _____ is the abnormal condition of having a thrombus.

5.28. The _____ are the blood cells involved in defending the body against infective organisms and foreign substances.

5.29. The hardening and narrowing of the arteries caused by a buildup of cholesterol plaque on the interior walls of the arteries is known as _____.

5.30. A/An _____ is a foreign object, such as a blood clot, quantity of air or gas, or a bit of tissue or tumor, that is circulating in the blood.

Matching Medical Terms and Definitions #1

Write the correct answer in the middle column.

Definitions	Correct Answer	Possible Answers
5.31. oxygen-carrying pigment	_____	anticoagulant
5.32. prevents new clots from forming	_____	beta-blocker
5.33. red blood cells	_____	erythrocytes
5.34. slows the heartbeat	_____	hemoglobin
5.35. stop or control bleeding	_____	hemostasis

Word Surgery

Divide these terms into word parts, in the proper sequence, on the lines provided to create the answer to the question. Use a slash (/) to indicate a combining form. Use a hyphen to indicate a prefix or suffix. (You may not need all of the lines provided.)

5.36. A carotid **endarterectomy** is the surgical removal of the lining of a portion of a clogged carotid artery leading to the brain.

_____   _____   _____   _____

5.37. **Cardiomyopathy** is the term used to describe all diseases of the heart muscle.

_____   _____   _____   _____

5.38. A **coronary thrombosis** is damage to the heart muscle caused by a thrombus blocking a coronary artery.

_____   _____   _____   _____

5.39. Blood **dyscrasia** is any pathologic condition of the cellular elements of the blood.

_____   _____   _____   _____

5.40. **Thrombocytopenia** is a condition in which there is an abnormally small number of platelets circulating in the blood.

_____   _____   _____   _____

Fill in the Blank #2

5.41. The peripheral arterial occlusive disease in which intermittent attacks are triggered by cold or stress is known as _____.

5.42. The type of vasculitis that can cause headaches, visual impairment, and jaw pain is known as _____.

5.43. The condition in which venous circulation is inadequate due to partial vein blockage or leakage of venous valves is known as chronic _____ (CVI).

5.44. In a/an _____ test, the flow of blood through the heart during activity is evaluated by injecting thallium into the bloodstream.

5.45. The diagnostic procedure in which a catheter is passed into a vein or artery and then guided into the heart is known as _____.

Multiple Choice

Select the correct answer and write it on the line provided.

5.46. The rapid, irregular, and useless contractions of the ventricles is known as ventricular _____.

    fibrillation   tachycardia

5.47. The condition known as _____ fibrillation occurs when the normal rhythmic contractions of the atria are replaced by rapid irregular twitching of the muscular heart wall.

    atrial   ventricular

5.48. The term _____ describes a group of cardiac disabilities resulting from an insufficient supply of oxygenated blood to the heart.

    angina pectoris   ischemic heart disease

5.49. An event in which the heart abruptly stops or develops a very abnormal arrhythmia that prevents it from pumping blood is known as a/an _____.

    cardiac arrest   ventricular tachycardia

5.50. A/An _____ is the occlusion of one or more coronary arteries caused by plaque buildup.

    coronary thrombosis   myocardial infarction

Word Construction #2

Use these word parts to construct the term that answers the following questions. Combining vowels are used in the term only when necessary. The answer includes the term (plus the appropriate word parts). For example: *hepatitis* (hepat, -itis).

angi/o	brady-	card/o	cardi/o	electr/o	embol/o	endo-
-gram	-graphy	hem/o	-ia	-ism	-itis	-ium
-lytic	-osis	peri-	phleb/o	-plasty	tachy-	thromb/o

5.51. A/An _____ is a record of the electrical activity of the myocardium.

5.52. The condition known as _____ anemia is characterized by an inadequate number of circulating red blood cells.

5.53. An abnormally rapid resting heart rate is known as _____.

5.54. The technique of mechanically widening a narrowed or obstructed blood vessel is known as a/an _____.

5.55. A/An _____ dissolves or causes a thrombus to break up.

5.56. The _____ surrounds and encloses the heart.

5.57. The inflammation of a vein is known as _____.

5.58. A/An _____ is the sudden blockage of a blood vessel by an embolus.

5.59. Inflammation of the inner lining of the heart is known as _____.

5.60. The term _____ describes an abnormally slow resting heart rate.

Matching Medical Terms and Definitions #2

Write the correct answer in the middle column.

Definitions	Correct Answer	Possible Answers
5.61. abnormally swollen veins	_____	aneurysm
5.62. balloon-like enlargement	_____	cholesterol
5.63. infection caused by bacteria in the blood	_____	diuretic
5.64. fatty substance found in the blood	_____	septicemia
5.65. medication to stimulate the kidneys	_____	varicose veins

Fill in the Blank #3

5.66. The use of electrical shock to restore the heart's normal rhythm is known as _____.

5.67. The condition of episodes of severe chest pain due to inadequate blood flow to the myocardium is known as _____.

5.68. A/An _____ is the blocking of an artery by a thrombus.

5.69. The blood disorder characterized by anemia in which the red blood cells are larger than normal is known as _____.

5.70. The term _____ describes damage to the heart muscle caused by a thrombus blocking a coronary artery.

5.71. The condition known as _____ is caused by a lack of a protein intrinsic factor.

5.72. The genetic disorder that causes abnormal hemoglobin is known as _____.

5.73. The condition known as _____ is characterized by an absence of all formed blood elements.

5.74. The loss of the normal rhythm of the heartbeat is known as _____.

5.75. The occurrence of rapid, irregular, and useless contractions of the ventricles is known as _____.

CHAPTER 5 CROSSWORD PUZZLE

The answers for this puzzle are located at the back of this workbook on page 97.

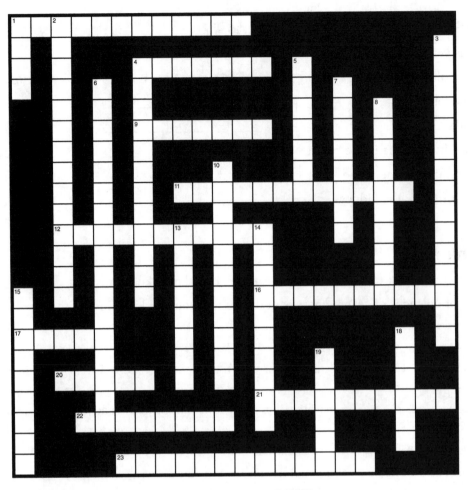

ACROSS

1. Inflammation of the inner lining of the heart
4. A foreign object circulating in the blood
9. Combining form meaning clot
11. A drug that dissolves a thrombus
12. Abnormally fast resting heart rate
16. To control bleeding
17. Combining form meaning white
20. Combining form meaning aorta
21. Myocardial _____ , heart attack
22. The blockage of a vessel by an embolus
23. Medication that slows blood coagulation

DOWN

1. Suffix meaning blood or blood condition
2. Electric shock used to restore the heart's rhythm
3. Hardening of the arteries due to a build-up of cholesterol plaque
4. Mature red blood cells
5. Combining form meaning artery or arteries
6. Record of electrical activity of the heart
7. Balloon-like enlargement of an artery wall
8. Severe infection caused by the presence of bacteria in the blood
10. An abnormally slow resting heart rate
13. Anemia marked by an absence of all formed blood elements
14. Loss of normal heartbeat rhythm
15. Inflammation of a vein
18. Episodes of severe chest pain
19. Suffix meaning a mixture or blending

The Lymphatic and Immune Systems

Learning Exercises

Class _____   Name _____

Matching Word Parts #1

Write the correct answer in the middle column.

Definition	Correct Answer	Possible Answers
6.1. cancerous	_____	carcin/o
6.2. flesh	_____	immun/o
6.3. pertaining to	_____	onc/o
6.4. protected, safe	_____	sarc/o
6.5. tumor	_____	-tic

Matching Word Parts #2

Write the correct answer in the middle column.

Definition	Correct Answer	Possible Answers
6.6. lymph	_____	-oma
6.7. lymph node	_____	neo-, ne/o
6.8. lymph vessel	_____	lymph/o
6.9. new	_____	lymphangi/o
6.10. tumor	_____	lymphaden/o

Matching Word Parts #3

Write the correct answer in the middle column.

Definition	Correct Answer	Possible Answers
6.11. against	_____	tox/o
6.12. eat, swallow	_____	splen/o
6.13. formative material of cells	_____	-plasm
6.14. spleen	_____	phag/o
6.15. poison	_____	anti-

Fill in the Blank #1

6.16. The term _____ is used to describe all lymphomas other than Hodgkin's lymphoma.

6.17. A/An _____ occurs when the immune response is compromised.

6.18. The form of breast cancer that starts in the milk duct, breaks through the wall of that duct, and invades the fatty breast tissue is known as _____ carcinoma.

6.19. A/An _____, which is also known as the immune reaction, involves binding antigens to antibodies.

6.20. The _____ syndrome, which is commonly known as AIDS, is the most advanced and fatal stage of an HIV infection.

Word Construction #1

Use these word parts to construct the term that answers the following questions. Combining vowels are used in the term only when necessary. The answer includes the term (plus the appropriate word parts). For example: *hepatitis* (hepat, -itis).

anti-	carcin/o	cyt/o	-edema	-ic	immun/o	-itis
lymph/o	lymphaden/o	lymphangi/o	megal/o	my/o	myc/o	-oma
-osis	oste/o	-pathy	sarc/o	tox/o	-us	vir/o

6.21. A/An _____ is a malignant tumor derived from muscle tissue.

6.22. The medical term meaning an inflammation of the lymph nodes is _____; however, the condition is commonly known as swollen glands.

6.23. A/An _____ drug is a medication that kills or damages cells.

6.24. Any disease process affecting a lymph node or nodes is described as being _____.

6.25. A/An _____ (CMV) is a member of the herpes virus family that causes a variety of diseases.

6.26. A benign tumor made up of muscle tissue is known as a/an _____.

6.27. A/An _____ is a malignant tumor that occurs in epithelial tissue.

6.28. A benign tumor formed by an abnormal collection of lymphatic vessels due to a congenital malformation of the lymphatic system is known as a/an _____.

6.29. A/An _____ is a malignant tumor usually involving the upper shaft of long bones, the pelvis, or knee.

6.30. Swelling due to an abnormal accumulation of lymph fluid within the tissues is known as _____.

Matching Microorganisms and Their Names

Write the correct answer in the middle column.

Definitions	Correct Answer	Possible Answers
6.31. bacteria that form chains	_____	bacilli
6.32. bacteria that form clusters	_____	rickettsia
6.33. rod-shaped bacteria	_____	spirochetes
6.34. small bacteria that live in lice	_____	staphylococci
6.35. spiral-shaped bacteria	_____	streptococci

Word Surgery

Divide these terms into word parts, in the proper sequence, on the lines provided to create the answer to the question. Use a slash (/) to indicate a combining form. Use a hyphen to indicate a prefix or suffix. (You may not need all of the lines provided.)

6.36. **A macrophage** is a type of white blood cell that surrounds and kills invading cells.

_____ _____ _____ _____

6.37. The spleen has the **hemolytic** function of destroying worn-out red blood cells and releasing their hemoglobin for reuse.

_____ _____ _____ _____

6.38. **Mammography** is a radiographic examination of the breasts to detect the presence of tumors or precancerous cells.

_____ _____ _____ _____

6.39. **Lymphoma** is a general term applied to malignancies affecting lymphoid tissues.

_____ _____ _____ _____

6.40. **Splenomegaly** is an abnormal enlargement of the spleen.

_____ _____ _____ _____

Fill in the Blank #2

6.41. The parasite _____ is most commonly transmitted from pets to humans by contact with contaminated feces.

6.42. A/An _____ is caused by a pathogen that does not normally produce an illness in healthy humans.

6.43. The group of proteins released primarily by the T cells, which act as signals to begin the immune response, are known as _____.

6.44. Commonly known as shingles, _____ is an acute viral infection characterized by painful skin eruptions that follow the underlying route of an inflamed nerve.

6.45. The family of proteins produced by the T cells whose specialty is fighting viruses by slowing or stopping their multiplication is known as _____.

Multiple Choice

Select the correct answer and write it on the line provided.

6.46. To _____ is the process by which cancer spreads from one place to another.

metastasis   metastasize

6.47. A _____ is a new cancer site that results from the spreading process.

metastasis   metastasize

6.48. The condition known as _____ is a viral infection characterized by a low-grade fever, swollen glands, inflamed eyes, and a fine, pink rash.

rabies   rubella

6.49. A systemic reaction, which is also described as _____, is a severe response to an allergen.

anaphylaxis   autoimmune disorder

6.50. The term _____ describes a malignant tumor in its original position that has not yet disturbed or invaded the surrounding tissues.

carcinoma in situ   ductal carcinoma

Word Construction #2

Use these word parts to construct the term that answers the following questions. Combining vowels are used in the term only when necessary. The answer includes the term (plus the appropriate word parts). For example: *hepatitis* (hepat, -itis).

-al	anti-	bio	brachy-	carcin/o	-cytes	fung/o
-ic	lymph/o	-oma	sarc/o	tele-	-therapy	-tic

6.51. A/An _____ is an agent that destroys or inhibits the growth of fungi.

6.52. Radiation therapy administered at a distance from the body is known as _____.

6.53. The term _____ describes white blood cells that are formed in bone marrow as stem cells.

6.54. A/An _____ is a medication that is capable of inhibiting the growth of or killing pathogenic bacterial microorganisms.

6.55. A malignant tumor that arises from connective tissues, including hard tissues, soft tissues, and liquid tissues, is known as a/an _____.

Fill in the Blank #3

6.56. Also known as anaphylactic shock, a _____ reaction is a severe response to an allergen.

6.57. The condition known as _____, or chickenpox, is caused by a herpes virus and is highly contagious.

6.58. The Epstein-Barr virus causes _____ and is characterized by fever, a sore throat, and enlarged lymph nodes.

6.59. The disease known as _____ is caused by a parasite that lives in certain mosquitoes and is transferred to humans by the bite of an infected mosquito.

6.60. The diagnostic test performed to detect damage or malformations of the lymphatic vessels is known as _____.

Matching Medical Terms and Definitions

Write the correct answer in the middle column.

Definitions	Correct Answer	Possible Answers
6.61. acute viral infection	_____	allergen
6.62. yeast infection	_____	antibody
6.63. disease-fighting protein	_____	candidiasis
6.64. lives on or within another organism	_____	parasite
6.65. produces an allergic reaction	_____	rabies

Fill in the Blank #4

6.66. A disease treatment that involves either stimulating or repressing the immune response is known as _____.

6.67. A/An _____ is any substance that the body regards as being foreign and includes viruses, bacteria, toxins, and transplanted tissues.

6.68. The group of proteins that normally circulate in the blood in an inactive form and are activated by contact with nonspecific antigens such as foreign blood cells or bacteria is known as _____.

6.69. _____ is distinguished from other lymphomas by the presence of large cancerous lymphocytes known as Reed-Sternberg cells.

6.70. The term _____ describes one-celled microscopic organisms. Most are not harmful to humans; however, some are pathogenic.

6.71. A/An _____ is any of a large group of diseases characterized by a condition in which the immune system produces antibodies to work against its own tissues.

6.72. Breast cancer at its earliest stage before the cancer has broken through the wall of the milk duct is known as _____ in situ.

6.73. The _____ virus, which is commonly known as HIV, is a bloodborne infection in which the virus damages or kills the cells of the immune system.

6.74. A/An _____ is a substance that prevents or reduces the body's normal immune response.

6.75. In the antigen–antibody response, _____ bind with specific antigens.

CHAPTER 6 CROSSWORD PUZZLE

The answers for this puzzle are located at the back of this workbook on page 98.

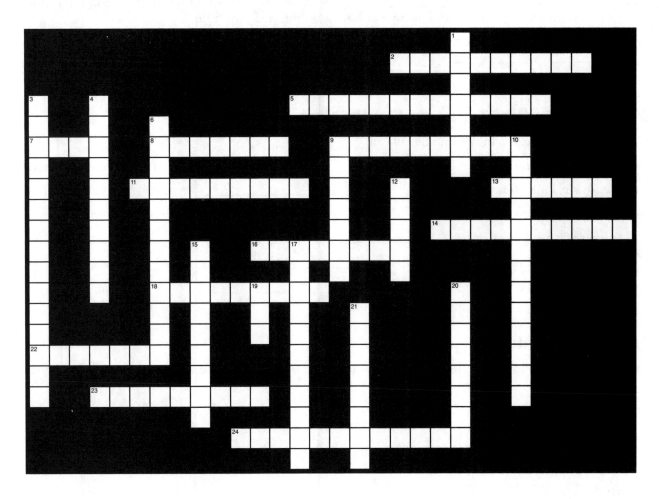

ACROSS

2. A new cancer site that results from the spreading process
5. Bacteria that form irregular groups or clusters resembling grapes
7. Combining form meaning poison
8. A malignant tumor that arises from connective tissue
9. An agent that destroys or inhibits the growth of fungi
11. Function that destroys worn-out red blood cells
13. Combining form meaning protection
14. Swelling due to an abnormal accumulation of lymph fluid within the tissues
16. Response to an allergen, _____ reaction
18. A drug that kills or damages cells
22. Also known as German measles
23. Also known as chickenpox
24. An abnormal enlargement of the spleen

DOWN

1. Combining form meaning cancerous
3. A type of herpesvirus also known as CMV
4. Malignant tumor derived from muscle tissue
6. A malignant tumor of bone
9. Any substance that the body regards as being foreign
10. Also known as swollen glands
12. Combining form meaning flesh
15. Proteins released primarily by the T cells
17. Spiral-shaped bacteria
19. Suffix meaning tumor
20. A disease-fighting protein created by the immune system
21. A malignancy that develops in the lymphatic system

The Respiratory System

Learning Exercises

Class _____   Name _____

Matching Word Parts #1

Write the correct answer in the middle column.

Definition	Correct Answer	Possible Answers
7.1. nose	_____	-thorax
7.2. breathing	_____	pneum/o
7.3. bronchus	_____	-pnea
7.4. chest	_____	nas/o
7.5. lung	_____	bronch/o

Matching Word Parts #2

Write the correct answer in the middle column.

Definition	Correct Answer	Possible Answers
7.6. larynx	_____	laryng/o
7.7. lung	_____	ox/o
7.8. pleura	_____	pharyng/o
7.9. oxygen	_____	pleur/o
7.10. pharynx	_____	pulmon/o

Matching Word Parts #3

Write the correct answer in the middle column.

Definition	Correct Answer	Possible Answers
7.11. sinus	_____	phon/o
7.12. sleep	_____	sinus/o
7.13. to breathe	_____	somn/o
7.14. voice or sound	_____	spir/o
7.15. windpipe	_____	trache/o

Fill in the Blank #1

7.16. The _____ is the cavity located between the lungs.

7.17. A/An _____ pumps air or oxygen through a liquid medicine to turn it into a vapor.

7.18. An irregular pattern of breathing characterized by alternating rapid or shallow respiration followed by slower respiration or apnea is known as _____ respiration.

7.19. An acute respiratory syndrome in children and infants characterized by obstruction of the larynx, hoarseness, and a barking cough is known as _____.

7.20. The infectious disease caused by *Mycobacterium tuberculosis* is known as _____.

Word Construction #1

Use these word parts to construct the term that answers the following questions. Combining vowels are used in the term only when necessary. The answer includes the term (plus the appropriate word parts). For example: *hepatitis* (hepat, -itis).

bronch/o	capn/o	-ectomy	-emia	hyper-	hypo-	-ia	ox/o
-pnea	pneum/o	pneumon/o	-rrhagia	-rrhea	-scopy	-spasm	-thorax

7.21. The abnormal buildup of carbon dioxide in the blood is known as _____.

7.22. A/An _____ is the accumulation of air in the pleural space.

7.23. An excessive discharge of mucus from the bronchi is known as _____.

7.24. Breathing commonly associated with exertion that is deeper and more rapid than is normal at rest is known as a/an _____.

7.25. The visual examination of the bronchi using a bronchoscope is known as _____.

7.26. The term _____ describes the condition of having below-normal oxygen levels in the blood.

7.27. A/An _____ is the surgical removal of all or part of a lung.

7.28. The condition of having below-normal oxygen levels in the body tissues and cells is known as _____.

7.29. The condition of a contraction of the smooth muscle in the walls of the bronchi and bronchioles is known as a/an _____.

7.30. Shallow or slow respiration is known as _____.

Matching Medical Terms and Definitions #1

Write the correct answer in the middle column.

Definitions	Correct Answer	Possible Answers
7.31. inflammation of the sinuses	_____	epistaxis
7.32. nosebleed	_____	laryngectomy
7.33. pain in the pleura	_____	pertussis
7.34. surgical removal of the larynx	_____	pleurodynia
7.35. whooping cough	_____	sinusitis

Word Surgery

Divide these terms into word parts, in the proper sequence, on the lines provided to create the answer to the question. Use a slash (/) to indicate a combining form. Use a hyphen to indicate a prefix or suffix. (You may not need all of the lines provided.)

7.36. **Pneumoconiosis** is fibrosis of the lung tissues caused by dust in the lungs that usually develops after prolonged environmental or occupational contact.

_____   _____   _____   _____

7.37. **Polysomnography** is also known as a sleep study.

_____   _____   _____   _____

7.38. A pulse **oximeter** is an external monitor placed on the patient's finger or earlobe to measure the oxygen saturation level in the blood.

_____   _____   _____   _____

7.39. A **pulmonologist** specializes in diagnosing and treating diseases and disorders of the lungs and associated tissues.

_____   _____   _____   _____

7.40. **Anoxia** is the absence of oxygen from the body's tissues and organs.

_____   _____   _____   _____

Fill in the Blank #2

7.41. The condition in which the alveoli and air passages fill with pus and other liquid is known as _____.

7.42. The presence of pus in the pleural cavity between the layers of the pleural membrane is known as _____.

7.43. A/An _____ is a collection of pus within a body cavity.

7.44. The progressive loss of lung function that is characterized by a decrease in the total number of alveoli, the enlargement of the remaining alveoli, and the progressive destruction of the walls of the remaining alveoli is known as _____.

7.45. The condition known as _____ is an inflammation of the pleura that produces sharp chest pain with each breath.

Multiple Choice

Select the correct answer and write it on the line provided.

7.46. A _____ is usually an emergency procedure in which an incision is made into the trachea to gain access to the airway below a blockage.

     tracheostomy   tracheotomy

7.47. The condition known as _____ is a chronic allergic disorder characterized by episodes of severe breathing difficulty, coughing, and wheezing.

     apnea   asthma

7.48. The genetic disorder in which the lungs and pancreas are clogged with large quantities of abnormally thick mucus is known as _____.

     cystic fibrosis   diphtheria

7.49. Coughing up bloodstained sputum is known as _____.

     hemoptysis   hemothorax

7.50. The collapse of part or all of a lung by blockage of the air passages or pneumothorax is known as _____.

     anthracosis   atelectasis

Word Construction #2

Use these word parts to construct the term that answers the following questions. Combining vowels are used in the term only when necessary. The answer includes the term (plus the appropriate word parts). For example: *hepatitis* (hepat, -itis).

brady-	-centesis	cost/o	hem/o	-itis	laryng/o	-osis
-ostomy	-otomy	ox/y	pharyng/o	-plegia	-pnea	-scopy
-spasm	spir/o	tachy-	thor/a	thorac/o	-thorax	trache/o

7.51. A/An _____ is a collection of blood in the pleural cavity.

7.52. The surgical incision into the chest walls to open the pleural cavity is known as a/an _____.

7.53. The condition known as _____ is the sudden spasmodic closure of the larynx.

7.54. An abnormally slow rate of respiration, usually of less than 10 breaths per minute, is known as a/an _____.

7.55. The procedure known as _____ is the surgical puncture of the chest wall with a needle to obtain fluid from the pleural cavity.

7.56. A/An _____ is the visual examination of the larynx.

7.57. The medical term for the condition commonly known as a sore throat is _____.

7.58. An abnormally rapid rate of respiration, usually of more than 20 breaths per minute, is known as _____.

7.59. A/An _____ is the creation of a stoma into the trachea.

7.60. An inflammation of the larynx is known as _____.

Matching Medical Terms and Definitions #2

Write the correct answer in the middle column.

Definitions	Correct Answer	Possible Answers
7.61. any change in vocal quality	_____	aphonia
7.62. asbestos particles in the lungs	_____	asbestosis
7.63. bluish discoloration of the skin	_____	cyanosis
7.64. loss of the ability to produce normal speech	_____	dysphonia
7.65. shortness of breath	_____	dyspnea

Fill in the Blank #3

7.66. The disorder in which breathing repeatedly stops and starts during sleep is known as _____.

7.67. The recording device that measures the amount of air inhaled or exhaled is a/an _____.

7.68. A/An _____ is commonly known as cough medicine.

7.69. The condition that occurs when the body cannot get the air it needs to function is known as _____.

7.70. The condition known as _____ is an acute bacterial infection of the throat and upper respiratory tract that is now largely prevented through immunization.

7.71. The passage of a tube through the nose or mouth into the trachea to establish or maintain an open airway is known as _____ .

7.72. Also known as air sacs, the very small clusters found at the end of each bronchiole are called _____.

7.73. A/An _____ is a medication that expands the opening of the passages into the lungs.

7.74. A/An _____ specializes in the diagnosis and treatment of diseases and disorders of the ears, nose, throat, and related structures of the head and neck.

7.75. Thick mucus secreted by the tissues lining the respiratory passages is called _____.

CHAPTER 7 CROSSWORD PUZZLE

The answers for this puzzle are located at the back of this workbook on page 99.

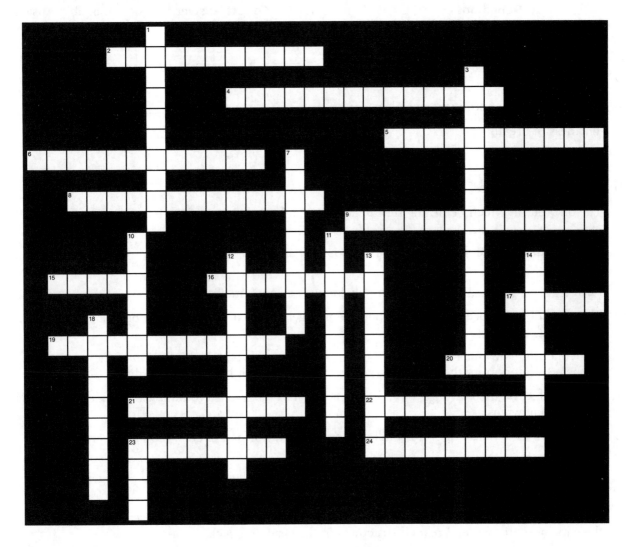

ACROSS

2. The collapse of part or all of a lung
4. Medication that expands the opening of the passages into the lungs
5. Inflammation of the pharynx
6. Sudden spasmodic closure of the larynx
8. Puncture of the chest wall with a needle to obtain fluid from the pleural cavity
9. Surgical removal of all or part of a lung
15. Childhood respiratory disease characterized by a barking cough
16. Having below normal oxygen level in the blood
17. Absence of spontaneous respiration
19. An accumulation of air in the pleural space causing the lung to not expand fully or to collapse
20. Difficult or labored breathing
21. An abnormally slow rate of respiration
22. Abnormally rapid respiratory rate
23. An inflammation of the pleura which produces sharp chest pain
24. Inflammation of the sinuses

DOWN

1. A collection of blood in the pleural cavity
3. Measures physiological activity during sleep
7. Nosebleed
10. A collection of pus in a body cavity
11. Coughing up blood
12. An abnormal build-up of carbon dioxide in the blood
13. Inflammation of the larynx
14. Shallow or slow respiration
18. Whooping cough
23. Suffix meaning breathing

The Digestive System

Learning Exercises

Class _____   Name _____

Matching Word Parts #1

Write the correct answer in the middle column.

Definition	Correct Answer	Possible Answers
8.1. anus	_____	an/o
8.2. anus and rectum	_____	chol/e
8.3. bile, gall	_____	col/o
8.4. colon	_____	-pepsia
8.5. digestion	_____	proct/o

Matching Word Parts #2

Write the correct answer in the middle column.

Definition	Correct Answer	Possible Answers
8.6. esophagus	_____	rect/o
8.7. gallbladder	_____	-lithiasis
8.8. liver	_____	hepat/o
8.9. presence of stones	_____	esophag/o
8.10. rectum	_____	cholecyst/o

Matching Word Parts #3

Write the correct answer in the middle column.

Definition	Correct Answer	Possible Answers
8.11. sigmoid colon	_____	-emesis
8.12. small intestine	_____	enter/o
8.13. stomach	_____	gastr/o
8.14. swallowing	_____	-phagia
8.15. vomiting	_____	sigmoid/o

Fill in the Blank #1

8.16. The term _____ describes a yellow discoloration of the skin, mucous membranes, and the eyes.

8.17. The condition of weighing two to three times, or more, than the ideal weight is known as _____.

8.18. _____ is a chronic autoimmune disorder that can occur any where in the digestive tract.

8.19. The condition of physical wasting away due to the loss of weight and muscle mass that occurs in patients with diseases such as advanced cancer or AIDS is known as _____.

8.20. The _____ is a laboratory test for hidden blood in the stools.

Word Construction #1

Use these word parts to construct the term that answers the following questions. Combining vowels are used in the term only when necessary. The answer includes the term (plus the appropriate word parts). For example: *hepatitis* (hepat, -itis).

aer/o	cholangi/o	cholecyst/o	choledoch/o	col/e	colon/o	dys-	-graphy
-itis	lith/o	-lithiasis	-ostomy	-otomy	-pepsia	-phagia	-scopy

8.21. The term _____ describes difficulty in swallowing.

8.22. The term _____ describes an inflammation of the gallbladder.

8.23. An acute infection of the bile duct is known as _____.

8.24. A/An _____ is the direct visual examination of the inner surface of the colon.

8.25. The medical term for the condition commonly known as indigestion is _____.

8.26. The term _____ describes a surgical creation of an opening between the colon and the body surface.

8.27. A/An _____ is a radiographic examination of the bile ducts.

8.28. The excessive swallowing of air while eating or drinking is known as _____.

8.29. The presence of gallstones in the gallbladder or bile ducts is known as _____.

8.30. A/An _____ is an incision into the common bile duct for the removal of gallstones.

Matching Medical Terms and Definitions #1

Write the correct answer in the middle column.

Definitions	Correct Answer	Possible Answers
8.31. mushroomlike growth	_____	aphthous ulcers
8.32. canker sores	_____	cheilosis
8.33. cold sores	_____	cirrhosis
8.34. disorder of the lips	_____	herpes labialis
8.35. degenerative disease of the liver	_____	polyp

Word Surgery

Divide these terms into word parts, in the proper sequence, on the lines provided to create the answer to the question. Use a slash (/) to indicate a combining form. Use a hyphen to indicate a prefi x or suffi x. (You may not need all of the lines provided.)

8.36. **Nasogastric** intubation is the placement of a feeding tube through the nose and into the stomach.

_____   _____   _____

8.37. **Gastroesophageal** reflux disease (GERD) is the upward flow of acid from the stomach into the esophagus.

_____   _____   _____

8.38. An **esophagogastroduodenoscopy** is an endoscopic procedure that allows direct visualization of the upper GI tract.

_____   _____   _____

8.39. **Leukoplakia** is an abnormal white lesion on the tongue or cheek.

_____   _____   _____

8.40. A **gastrostomy** tube is a surgically placed feeding tube from the exterior of the body into the stomach.

_____   _____   _____

Fill in the Blank #2

8.41. The term _____ describes a series of wavelike contractions of the smooth muscles in a single direction.

8.42. An excessive accumulation of fat in the body is known as _____.

8.43. The term _____ describes any restriction to the opening of the mouth caused by trauma, surgery, or radiation associated with the treatment of oral cancer.

8.44. The term _____ describes the act of belching or raising gas orally from the stomach.

8.45. Enlarged and swollen veins at the lower end of the esophagus are known as _____.

Multiple Choice

Select the correct answer and write it on the line provided.

8.46. The inflammation of one or more diverticula in the colon is known as _____.

   diverticulitis   diverticulosis

8.47. The term _____ describes the twisting of the intestine on itself that causes an obstruction.

   ileus   volvulus

8.48. The eating disorder characterized by frequent episodes of binge eating is known as _____ nervosa.

   anorexia   bulimia

8.49. The branch of medicine concerned with the prevention and control of obesity and associated diseases is known as _____.

   bariatrics   gastroenterology

8.50. The autoimmune disorder characterized by a severe reaction to gluten is known as _____.

   celiac disease   Crohn's disease

Word Construction #2

Use these word parts to construct the term that answers the following questions. Combining vowels are used in the term only when necessary. The answer includes the term (plus the appropriate word parts). For example: *hepatitis* (hepat, -itis).

-a	diverticul/o	-emesis	enter/o	hemat/o	hepat/o	hyper-
hypo-	-ia	-itis	melan/o	-osis	-ologist	proct/o
-rrhagia	-rrhea	-scopy	sigmoid/o	stom/o	stomat/o	xer/o

8.51. The presence of a number of diverticula in the colon is known as _____.

8.52. The passage of black, tarry, and foul-smelling stools is known as _____.

8.53. The lack of adequate saliva due to the absence of or diminished secretions by the salivary glands is known as _____.

8.54. The term _____ describes an inflammation of the small intestine.

8.55. The term _____ means vomiting blood.

8.56. An inflammation of the liver is known as _____.

8.57. A physician who specializes in disorders of the colon, rectum, and anus is known as a/an _____.

8.58. A/An _____ is the endoscopic examination of the interior of the rectum and sigmoid colon.

8.59. The term _____ describes an inflammation of the mucosa of the mouth.

8.60. Extreme, persistent vomiting that can cause dehydration is known as _____.

Matching Medical Terms and Definitions #2

Write the correct answer in the middle column.

Definitions	Correct Answer	Possible Answers
8.61. blockage of the intestine	_____	antiemetic
8.62. medication to prevent vomiting	_____	ascites
8.63. serous fluid in the peritoneal cavity	_____	ileus
8.64. swallowed food returned to the mouth	_____	peptic ulcers
8.65. sores on the membranes of the digestive system	_____	regurgitation

Fill in the Blank #3

8.66. The chronic condition in which repeated episodes of inflammation in the rectum and large intestine cause ulcers and irritation is known as _____.

8.67. A/An _____ is the establishment of an anastomosis between the upper portion of the stomach and the duodenum.

8.68. A/An _____ is a surgical connection between two hollow or tubular structures.

8.69. The condition in which a portion of the stomach protrudes upward through an opening in the diaphragm is known as a/an _____.

8.70. The surgical repair of a cleft palate or cleft lip is called _____.

8.71. A/An _____ is the protrusion of a small loop of bowel through a weak place in the lower abdominal wall.

8.72. The infectious disease of the intestine caused by the bacterium *Salmonella,* and transmitted by food that is contaminated by feces, is known as _____.

8.73. The eating disorder characterized by a false perception of body appearance is known as _____.

8.74. The rumbling noise caused by the movement of gas in the intestine is known as _____.

8.75. A/An _____ is the surgical removal of the gallbladder.

CHAPTER 8 CROSSWORD PUZZLE

The answers for this puzzle are located at the back of this workbook on page 100.

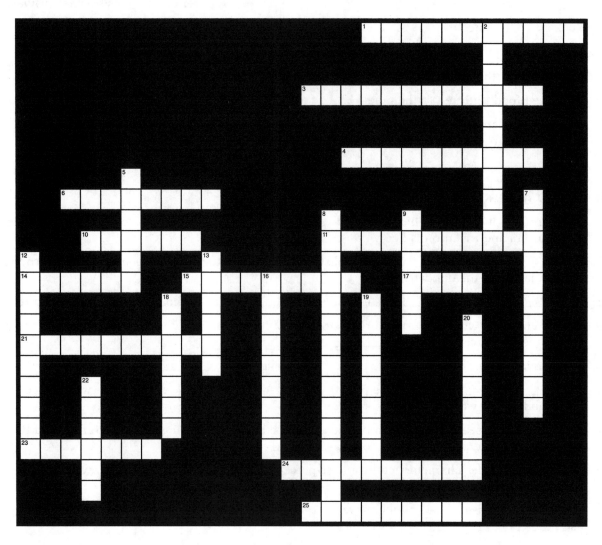

ACROSS

1. Wave-like contractions that move food through the digestive system
3. Surgical repair of a cleft palate
4. Also known as dry mouth
6. A yellow discoloration of the skin, mucous membranes, and the eyes
10. Also known as vomiting
11. Extreme, persistent vomiting
14. Combining form meaning liver
15. Test also known as the fecal occult blood test
17. Combining form meaning colon
21. The act of belching
23. An excessive accumulation of body fat
24. Inflammation of the mucosa of the mouth
25. Difficulty in swallowing

DOWN

2. A surgical connection between two hollow or tubular structures
5. Combining form meaning small intestine
7. A _____ tube is an external feeding tube
8. Surgical removal of the gallbladder
9. Combining form meaning rectum
12. Combining form meaning gallbladder
13. The passage of black, tarry stools
16. A chronic degenerative disease of the liver
18. Restriction of the opening of the mouth
19. Also known as indigestion
20. Twisting of the intestine on itself
22. Suffix meaning digestion

The Urinary System

Learning Exercises

Class _____   Name _____

Matching Word Parts #1

Write the correct answer in the middle column.

Definition	Correct Answer	Possible Answers
9.1. bladder	_____	-cele
9.2. complete, through	_____	cyst/o
9.3. enlargement, stretching	_____	dia-
9.4. glomerulus	_____	-ectasis
9.5. hernia, tumor, cyst	_____	glomerul/o

Matching Word Parts #2

Write the correct answer in the middle column.

Definition	Correct Answer	Possible Answers
9.6. urine, urinary tract	_____	ur/o
9.7. kidney	_____	-pexy
9.8. setting free, separation	_____	nephr/o
9.9. stone	_____	-lysis
9.10. surgical fixation	_____	lith/o

Matching Word Parts #3

Write the correct answer in the middle column.

Definition	Correct Answer	Possible Answers
9.11. renal pelvis	_____	-uria
9.12. to crush	_____	urethr/o
9.13. ureter	_____	ureter/o
9.14. urethra	_____	-tripsy
9.15. urination, urine	_____	pyel/o

Fill in the Blank #1

9.16. The progressive loss of renal function over months or years is known as _____.

9.17. A/An _____ tumor is a malignant tumor of the kidney that occurs in young children.

9.18. The term _____ describes the removal of a body part or the destruction of its function.

9.19. The procedure to remove waste products from the blood of a patient whose kidneys no longer function is known as _____.

9.20. The condition known as _____ bladder is a urinary problem caused by interference with the normal nerve pathways associated with urination.

Word Construction #1

Use these word parts to construct the term that answers the following questions. Combining vowels are used in the term only when necessary. The answer includes the term (plus the appropriate word parts). For example: *hepatitis* (hepat, -itis).

-ectasis	-emia	-itis	-lith	-otomy	-pexy
-rrhagia	-rrhaphy	-stenosis	ur/o	ureter/o	urethr/o

9.21. A/An _____ is the surgical incision into the urethra for relief of a stricture.

9.22. The toxic condition resulting from renal failure in which urea is retained in the blood is known as _____.

9.23. The condition known as _____ is the narrowing of the urethra.

9.24. The surgical suturing of a ureter is known as _____.

9.25. The term _____ describes bleeding from the urethra.

9.26. The distention of a ureter is described by the term _____.

9.27. The term _____ describes an inflammation of the urethra.

9.28. A/An _____ is a stone located anywhere along the ureter.

9.29. The surgical fixation of the urethra to nearby tissue is known as _____.

9.30. The discharge of blood from the ureter is known as _____.

Matching Medical Terms and Definitions #1

Write the correct answer in the middle column.

Definitions	Correct Answer	Possible Answers
9.31. absence of urine formation	_____	incontinence
9.32. filtering waste from the patient's blood	_____	hemodialysis
9.33. inability to control flow of body waste	_____	diuresis
9.34. increased output of urine	_____	catheterization
9.35. insertion of a tube into the bladder	_____	anuria

Word Surgery

Divide these terms into word parts, in the proper sequence, on the lines provided to create the answer to the question. Use a slash (/) to indicate a combining form. Use a hyphen to indicate a prefix or suffix. (You may not need all of the lines provided.)

9.36. Voiding **cystourethrography** is the use of a fluoroscope to examine the flow of urine.

_____   _____   _____   _____

9.37. An intravenous **pyelogram** is a radiographic study of the kidneys and ureters.

_____   _____   _____   _____

9.38. A **vesicovaginal** fistula is an abnormal opening between the bladder and vagina that allows the constant flow of urine from the bladder into the vagina.

_____   _____   _____   _____

9.39. A voiding **cystourethrography** is a diagnostic procedure to examine the flow of urine from the bladder and through the urethra.

_____   _____   _____   _____

9.40. **Polycystic** kidney disease is a genetic disorder characterized by the growth of numerous fluid-filled cysts in the kidneys.

_____   _____   _____   _____

Fill in the Blank #2

9.41. A/An _____ is performed by making a small incision in the back and inserting a nephroscope to crush and remove a kidney stone.

9.42. The medical term _____ is commonly known as bed-wetting.

9.43. Benign _____ (BPH) is an abnormal enlargement of the prostate gland that occurs most often in men over 50 years old.

9.44. Placement of a catheter into the bladder through a small incision made through the abdominal wall just above the pubic bone is known as _____.

9.45. _____ is a condition in which very high levels of protein are lost in the urine and abnormally low levels of protein are present in the blood.

Multiple Choice

Select the correct answer and write it on the line provided.

9.46. The presence of abnormally low concentrations of protein in the blood is known
as _____.

   hyperproteinuria   hypoproteinemia

9.47. The condition known as _____ is the suppuration of pus from the kidney.

   nephroptosis   nephropyosis

9.48. In _____, the lining of the peritoneal cavity acts as the filter to remove waste from
the blood.

   hemodialysis   peritoneal dialysis

9.49. In the male with _____, the urethral opening is on the undersurface of the penis.

   epispadias   hypospadias

9.50. The condition of having symptoms resulting from obstruction of the urethra due to benign prostatic
hypertrophy is known as _____.

   prostatism   prostatitis

Word Construction #2

Use these word parts to construct the term that answers the following questions. Combining vowels are
used in the term only when necessary. The answer includes the term (plus the appropriate word parts).
For example: *hepatitis* (hepat, -itis).

-emia	en-	glomerul/o	hydro-	hyper-	-itis
lith/o	nephr/o	noct/o	-osis	-otomy	-plasty
protein/o	-ptosis	pyel/o	-uresis	-ureter	-uria

9.51. The dilation of one or both kidneys is known as _____.

9.52. The term _____ describes the prolapse of a kidney.

9.53. A/An _____ is a surgical incision into the renal pelvis.

9.54. The term _____ describes the involuntary discharge of urine.

9.55. The kidney disease that causes red blood cells and proteins to leak into the urine is known
as _____.

9.56. A/An _____ is a surgical incision for the removal of a stone from the bladder.

9.57. The surgical repair of the renal pelvis is known as a/an _____.

9.58. The condition known as _____ is the distention of the ureter with urine that cannot flow because the ureter is blocked.

9.59. Abnormally high concentrations of protein in the urine is known as _____.

9.60. The term _____ describes excessive urination during the night.

Matching Medical Terms and Definitions #2

Write the correct answer in the middle column.

Definitions	Correct Answer	Possible Answers
9.61. bladder inflammation	_____	cystoscopy
9.62. fallen bladder	_____	cystopexy
9.63. stone in the bladder	_____	cystolith
9.64. surgical fixation of the bladder	_____	cystocele
9.65. visual examination of bladder interior	_____	cystitis

Fill in the Blank #3

9.66. The term _____ describes a chronic inflammation within the walls of the bladder.

9.67. The destruction of stones with the use of high-energy ultrasonic waves traveling through water or gel is known as _____ (ESWL).

9.68. In the female with _____, the urethral opening is in the region of the clitoris.

9.69. The term _____ means scanty urination.

9.70. The genetic disorder characterized by the growth of numerous fluid-filled cysts in the kidneys is known as _____ kidney disease (PKD).

9.71. The term _____ means excessive urination.

9.72. The establishment of an opening from the pelvis of the kidney to the exterior of the body is known as a/an _____.

9.73. The term _____ describes the presence of stones in the kidney.

9.74. The term meaning any disease of the kidney is _____.

9.75. The freeing of a kidney from adhesions is _____.

CHAPTER 9 CROSSWORD PUZZLE

The answers for this puzzle are located at the back of this workbook on page 101.

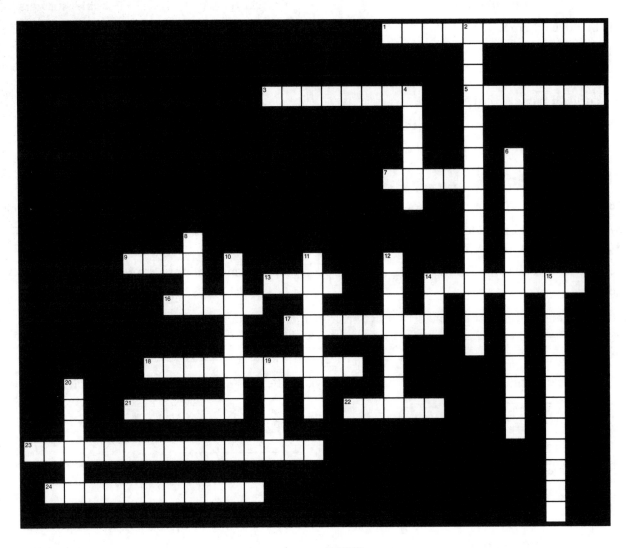

ACROSS

1. Incision into the urethra for relief of a stricture
3. Excessive urination during the night
5. Suffix meaning enlargement or stretching
7. Combining form meaning stone
9. Suffix meaning hernia, tumor, or swelling
13. Suffix meaning urine
14. Increased output of urine
16. Combining form meaning renal pelvis
17. Scanty urination
18. Freeing a kidney from adhesions
21. Also known as uremic poisoning
22. Combining form meaning bladder
23. The presence of stones in the kidney
24. Surgical repair of the ureter and renal pelvis

DOWN

2. Abnormally high concentrations of protein in the urine
4. The absence of urine formation by the kidneys
6. The dilation of one or both kidneys
8. Suffix meaning surgical fixation
10. Excessive urination
11. Procedure to replace kidney function
12. Nocturnal_____is also known as bed-wetting
14. Prefix meaning complete or through
15. The inability to control the excretion of urine and feces
19. Suffix meaning separation
20. Suffix meaning to crush

The Nervous System

Learning Exercises

Class _____   Name _____

Matching Word Parts #1

Write the correct answer in the middle column.

Definition	Correct Answer	Possible Answers
10.1. abnormal fear	_____	caus/o
10.2. membranes, meninges	_____	contus/o
10.3. brain	_____	encephal/o
10.4. bruise	_____	mening/o
10.5. burning sensation	_____	-phobia

Matching Word Parts #2

Write the correct answer in the middle column.

Definition	Correct Answer	Possible Answers
10.6. feeling	_____	cerebr/o
10.7. having an affinity for	_____	esthet/o
10.8. cerebrum, brain	_____	neur/o
10.9. mind	_____	psych/o
10.10. nerve, nerves	_____	-tropic

Matching Word Parts #3

Write the correct answer in the middle column.

Definition	Correct Answer	Possible Answers
10.11. recording an image	_____	concuss/o
10.12. sensation, feeling	_____	-esthesia
10.13. shaken together	_____	-graphy
10.14. spinal cord (bone marrow)	_____	myel/o
10.15. nerve root	_____	radicul/o

Fill in the Blank #1

10.16. The _____ syndrome (GBS), which is also known as infectious polyneuritis, is characterized by rapidly worsening muscle weakness that can lead to temporary paralysis.

10.17. The anxiety disorder characterized by recurrent unwanted thoughts and/or impulses to act is known as a/an _____ disorder.

10.18. The term _____ disorder (PTSD) may develop after an event during which the person felt intense fear, helplessness, or horror.

10.19. The results of a child being violently shaken by someone are known as _____ syndrome, and this can cause brain injury, paralysis, or death.

10.20. The psychotic disorder known as _____ is usually characterized by withdrawal from reality, illogical patterns of thinking, delusions, and varying degrees of other emotional, behavioral, or intellectual disturbances.

Word Construction #1

Use these word parts to construct the term that answers the following questions. Combining vowels are used in the term only when necessary. The answer includes the term (plus the appropriate word parts). For example: *hepatitis* (hepat, -itis).

ad-	-algia	an-	caus/o	cephal/o	-dynia	ech/o
electr/o	encephal/o	esthet/o	-gram	-graphy	hydr/o	-ia
-ic	-ism	-ist	-itis	mening/o	myel/o	-us

10.21. A/An _____ is the medication used to induce anesthesia.

10.22. The condition in which excess cerebrospinal fluid accumulates in the brain is known as _____.

10.23. The condition known as _____ is an inflammation of the brain.

10.24. A/An _____ is a radiography study of the spinal cord using a contrast medium.

10.25. The process of recording the electrical activity of the brain through the use of electrodes attached to the scalp is known as _____.

10.26. An inflammation of the meninges of the brain and spinal cord is known as _____.

10.27. The condition known as _____ is persistent, severe burning pain that usually follows an injury to a sensory nerve.

10.28. The use of ultrasound imaging to create a detailed visual image of the brain is known as _____.

10.29. A/An _____ specializes in administering anesthesia but is not a physician.

10.30. The condition known as _____ is an inflammation of the spinal cord.

Matching Medical Terms and Definitions #1

Write the correct answer in the middle column.

Definitions	Correct Answer	Possible Answers
10.31. difficulty developing normal relationships	_____	autism
10.32. deep state of unconsciousness	_____	cognition
10.33. fainting	_____	coma
10.34. recurrent episodes of seizures	_____	epilepsy
10.35. thinking, learning, and memory	_____	syncope

Word Surgery

Divide these terms into word parts, in the proper sequence, on the lines provided to create the answer to the question. Use a slash (/) to indicate a combining form. Use a hyphen to indicate a prefix or suffix. (You may not need all of the lines provided.)

10.36. The condition of abnormal and excessive sensitivity to touch, pain, or other sensory stimuli is known as **hyperesthesia.**

_____   _____   _____   _____

10.37. Cervical **radiculopathy** is nerve pain caused by pressure on the spinal nerve roots in the neck region.

_____   _____   _____   _____

10.38. Carotid **ultrasonography** is an ultrasound study of the carotid artery.

_____   _____   _____   _____

10.39. A cerebral **contusion** is bruising of brain tissue as a result of a head injury.

_____   _____   _____   _____

10.40. **Paresthesia** refers to a burning or prickling sensation that is usually felt in the hands, arms, legs, or feet.

_____   _____   _____   _____

Fill in the Blank #2

10.41. A/An _____, which is the most common type of stroke in older people, occurs when the flow of blood to the brain is blocked.

10.42. The chemical substances that make it possible for messages to cross from the synapse of a neuron to the target receptor are known as _____.

10.43. _____ is a chronic, degenerative central nervous disorder characterized by fine muscle tremors, rigidity, and a slow or shuffling gait.

10.44. A/An _____ is a condition in which an individual acts as if he or she has a physical or mental illness when he or she is not really sick.

10.45. _____ is characterized by vomiting and confusion, and sometimes follows a viral illness in which the child was treated with aspirin.

Multiple Choice

Select the correct answer and write it on the line provided.

10.46. A _____ is a violent shaking up or jarring of the brain.

concussion   contusion

10.47. The lowered level of consciousness marked by listlessness, drowsiness, and apathy is known as _____.

lethargy   stupor

10.48. The term _____ describes an abnormal fear of being in small or enclosed spaces.

acrophobia   claustrophobia

10.49. A/An _____ is a sensory perception that is experienced in the absence of an external stimulation.

delusion   hallucination

10.50. A _____ is a collection of blood trapped in the tissues of the brain.

cerebral contusion   cranial hematoma

10.51. A/An _____ is an unexpected, sudden experience of fear in the absence of danger accompanied by physical symptoms.

anxiety disorder   panic attack

10.52. The fear that one has a serious illness despite appropriate medical evaluation and reassurance is known as _____.

delusion   hypochondriasis

10.53. _____ is the temporary paralysis of the seventh cranial nerve that causes paralysis of only the affected side of the face.

Bell's palsy   Trigeminal neuralgia

10.54. A/An _____ stroke occurs when a blood vessel in the brain leaks.

hemorrhagic   ischemic

10.55. The progressive autoimmune disorder characterized by inflammation that causes demyelination of the myelin sheath is known as _____.

Alzheimer's disease   multiple sclerosis

Fill in the Blank #3

10.56. _____ is a group of disorders involving the parts of the brain that control thought, memory, and language.

10.57. Inflammation of the sciatic nerve that results in pain, burning, and tingling along the course of the affected nerve is known as _____.

10.58. The condition known as _____ is characterized by severe lightning-like pain due to an inflammation of the fifth cranial nerve.

10.59. A/An _____ is a false personal belief that is maintained despite obvious proof or evidence to the contrary.

10.60. The _____ is the thick, tough, outermost membrane of the meninges.

Matching Medical Terms and Definitions #2

Write the correct answer in the middle column.

Definitions	Correct Answer	Possible Answers
10.61. decline in mental abilities	_____	acrophobia
10.62. developmental reading disorder	_____	delirium
10.63. disorientation due to high fever	_____	dementia
10.64. excessive fear of high places	_____	dyslexia
10.65. electrical activity in the brain	_____	seizure

Fill in the Blank #4

10.66. The condition known as _____ (ALS) is a rapidly progressive neurological disease that attacks the nerve cells responsible for controlling voluntary muscles.

10.67. Mental conditions characterized by excessive, irrational dread of everyday situations are known as _____ disorders.

10.68. A/An _____ headache, which can be preceded by a warning aura, is characterized by throbbing pain on one side of the head.

10.69. The condition characterized by poor muscle control, spasticity, speech defects, and other neurologic deficiencies due to damage that affects the cerebrum is known as _____ (CP).

10.70. The disorder of the nerves that carry information to and from the brain and spinal cord is known as _____.

10.71. The regional anesthesia produced by injecting a local anesthetic into the epidural space of the lumbar or sacral region of the spine is known as _____.

10.72. The disorder involving sudden and severe mental changes or seizures caused by abruptly stopping the use of alcohol is known as _____.

10.73. A/An _____ (CVA) is damage to the brain that occurs when the blood flow to the brain is disrupted because a blood vessel is either blocked or has ruptured.

10.74. A/An _____ is the congenital herniation of the meninges through a defect in the skull or spinal column.

10.75. The condition of _____ is a sleep disorder consisting of sudden and uncontrollable brief episodes of falling asleep during the day.

CHAPTER 10 CROSSWORD PUZZLE

The answers for this puzzle are located at the back of this workbook on page 102.

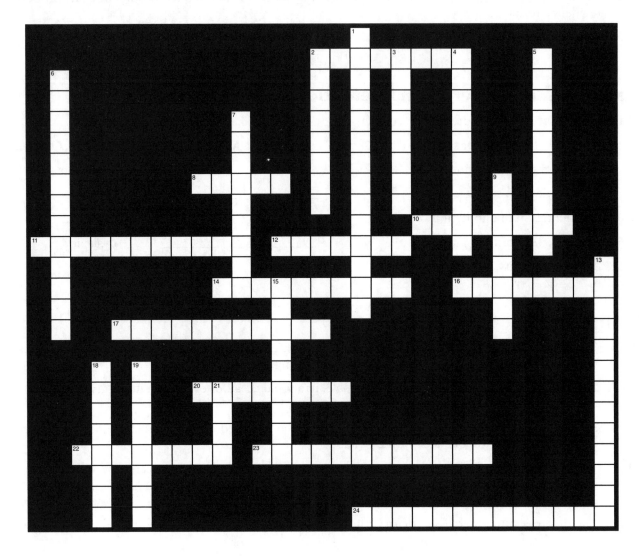

ACROSS

2. An acute condition of confusion and agitation
8. Combining form meaning spinal cord and bone marrow
10. Also known as a seizure disorder
11. An abnormal sensation such as burning or prickling
12. Also known as fainting
14. Violent shaking up or jarring of the brain
16. A lowered level of consciousness marked by listlessness and drowsiness
17. Type of stroke that is also known as a bleed
20. Inflammation of the sciatic nerve
22. A slowly progressive decline in mental abilities
23. Inflammation of the brain
24. A psychotic disorder characterized by withdrawal from reality

DOWN

1. Fear of being in small or enclosed spaces
2. A false personal belief
3. Combining form meaning root or nerve root
4. Inflammation of the meninges of the brain and spinal cord
5. Recurring episodes of falling asleep during the day
6. A sense perception with no basis in external stimulation
7. Combining form meaning brain
9. An inflammation of the spinal cord
13. A condition of excessive sensitivity to stimuli
15. Mental activities associated with thinking, learning, and memory
18. Suffix meaning sensation or feeling
19. Also known as a developmental reading disorder
21. Deep state of unconsciousness

Special Senses: The Eyes and Ears

Learning Exercises

Class _____   Name _____

Matching Word Parts #1

Write the correct answer in the middle column.

Definition	Correct Answer	Possible Answers
11.1. ear	_____	blephar/o
11.2. eye, vision	_____	ophthalm/o
11.3. eyelid	_____	-opia
11.4. old age	_____	ot/o
11.5. vision condition	_____	presby/o

Matching Word Parts #2

Write the correct answer in the middle column.

Definition	Correct Answer	Possible Answers
11.6. cornea, hard	_____	-cusis
11.7. eardrum	_____	irid/o
11.8. hearing	_____	kerat/o
11.9. iris	_____	myring/o
11.10. lens of eye	_____	phak/o

Matching Word Parts #3

Write the correct answer in the middle column.

Definition	Correct Answer	Possible Answers
11.11. eardrum	_____	tympan/o
11.12. eyes, vision	_____	trop/o
11.13. retina	_____	scler/o
11.14. turn	_____	retin/o
11.15. white of eye	_____	opt/o

Fill in the Blank #1

11.16. The condition known as _____ is a sense of whirling, dizziness, and the loss of balance that is often combined with nausea and vomiting.

11.17. A/An _____ is the loss of transparency of the lens, which causes a progressive loss of visual clarity.

11.18. The dilation of the pupil is known as _____.

11.19. A/An _____ is an electronic device that bypasses the damaged portions of the ear and directly stimulates the auditory nerve.

11.20. The term _____ means accessory structures of an organ.

Word Construction #1

Use these word parts to construct the term that answers the following questions. Combining vowels are used in the term only when necessary. The answer includes the term (plus the appropriate word parts). For example: *hepatitis* (hepat, -itis).

aden/o	-cusis	dacry/o	dipl/o	ec-	emmetr/o	en-	eso-
exo-	-ia	-ion	-itis	-opia	presby/o	scler/o	trop/o

11.21. The term _____ describes the condition of common changes in the eyes that occur with aging.

11.22. An inflammation of the lacrimal gland that can be caused by a bacterial, viral, or fungal infection is known as a/an _____.

11.23. The condition known as _____, or wall-eyes, is strabismus characterized by the outward deviation of one eye relative to the other.

11.24. The term _____ describes the perception of two images of a single object.

11.25. Strabismus characterized by an inward deviation of one eye or both eyes is known as _____.

11.26. The term _____ describes the gradual loss of sensorineural hearing that occurs as the body ages.

11.27. The turning outward of the edge of an eyelid is known as _____.

11.28. The term _____ describes an inflammation of the sclera.

11.29. The normal relationship between the refractive power of the eye and the shape of the eye that enables light rays to focus correctly on the retina is known as _____.

11.30. The term _____ describes the turning inward of the edge of an eyelid.

Matching Medical Terms and Definitions #1

Write the correct answer in the middle column.

Definitions	Correct Answer	Possible Answers
11.31. increased intraocular pressure	_____	amblyopia
11.32. inflammation of the conjunctiva	_____	chalazion
11.33. nodule or cyst on the upper eyelid	_____	conjunctivitis
11.34. partial loss of sight	_____	glaucoma
11.35. pus-filled lesion on the eyelid	_____	hordeolum

Word Surgery

Divide these terms into word parts, in the proper sequence, on the lines provided to create the answer to the question. Use a slash (/) to indicate a combining form. Use a hyphen to indicate a prefix or suffix. (You may not need all of the lines provided.)

11.36. **Barotrauma** is pressure-related ear discomfort that can be caused by pressure changes when the eustachian tube is blocked.

_____   _____   _____   _____

11.37. **Photophobia** means excessive sensitivity to light.

_____   _____   _____   _____

11.38. **Tarsorrhaphy** is the suturing together of the upper and lower eyelids.

_____   _____   _____   _____

11.39. An **optometrist** specializes in measuring the accuracy of vision to determine whether corrective lenses are needed.

_____   _____   _____   _____

11.40. Drying of the surfaces of the eye, including the conjunctiva, is known as **xerophthalmia**.

_____   _____   _____   _____

Fill in the Blank #2

11.41. The procedure known as _____ is a radiographic study of the blood vessels in the retina of the eye.

11.42. A/An _____ is used to treat open-angle glaucoma by creating openings in the trabecular meshwork to allow fluid to drain properly.

11.43. A/An _____ is a surgical procedure to treat myopia.

11.44. Swelling surrounding the eye or eyes is known as _____.

11.45. The condition known as _____ is swelling and inflammation of the optic nerve at the point of entrance into the eye through the optic disk.

Multiple Choice

Select the correct answer and write it on the line provided.

11.46. The term _____ describes the flow of pus from the ear.

   otomycosis   otopyorrhea

11.47. The condition known as _____ is an inflammation of the cornea.

   iritis   keratitis

11.48. The term _____ describes a defect in which light rays focus in front of the retina.

   hyperopia   myopia

11.49. The ankylosis of the bones of the middle ear resulting in a conductive hearing loss is known
   as _____.

   otorrhagia   otosclerosis

11.50. The surgical removal of the top portion of the stapes is known as a _____.

   labyrinthectomy   stapedectomy

Word Construction #2

Use these word parts to construct the term that answers the following questions. Combining vowels are used in the term only when necessary. The answer includes the term (plus the appropriate word parts). For example: *hepatitis* (hepat, -itis).

ametr/o	an-	anis/o	cor/o	-ectomy	hemi-
hyper-	-ia	-itis	labyrinth/o	mastoid/o	myc/o
myring/o	nyctal/o	-opia	-osis	ot/o	-rrhea

11.51. The term _____ means blindness in one half of the visual field.

11.52. Infectious _____ is a contagious inflammation that causes painful blisters on the eardrum.

11.53. A/An _____ is the surgical removal of mastoid cells.

11.54. The condition of _____ is commonly known as farsightedness.

11.55. The condition known as _____ is a fungal infection of the external auditory canal.

11.56. The term _____ describes any error of refraction in which images do not focus properly on the retina.

11.57. A/An _____ is the surgical removal of all or a portion of the labyrinth.

11.58. The condition in which the pupils are unequal in size is known as _____.

11.59. The term _____ describes discharge from the ear.

11.60. The condition in which an individual with normal daytime vision has difficulty seeing at night is known as _____.

Matching Medical Terms and Definitions #2

Write the correct answer in the middle column.

Definitions	Correct Answer	Possible Answers
11.61. eyes point in different directions	_____	astigmatism
11.62. measurement of intraocular pressure	_____	strabismus
11.63. ringing in the ears	_____	tinnitus
11.64. test for middle ear disorders	_____	tonometry
11.65. uneven curvature of the cornea	_____	tympanometry

Fill in the Blank #3

11.66. The removal of the vitreous fluid and its replacement with a clear solution is known as _____.

11.67. A/An _____ is the surgical incision in the eardrum to create an opening for the placement of tympanostomy tubes.

11.68. An inflammation of the middle ear is known as _____.

11.69. A/An _____ is the surgical removal of a portion of the tissue of the iris.

11.70. An involuntary, constant, rhythmic movement of the eyeball is known as _____.

11.71. A laser is used to reattach the detached area in a retinal detachment. This procedure is known as a/an _____ .

11.72. The visual examination of the fundus of the eye is known as _____.

11.73. The use of an audiometer to measure hearing acuity is known as _____.

11.74. An inflammation of the sclera is known as _____.

11.75. An inflammation of the uveal tract affecting primarily structures in the front of the eye is known as _____.

CHAPTER 11 CROSSWORD PUZZLE

The answers for this puzzle are located at the back of this workbook on page 103.

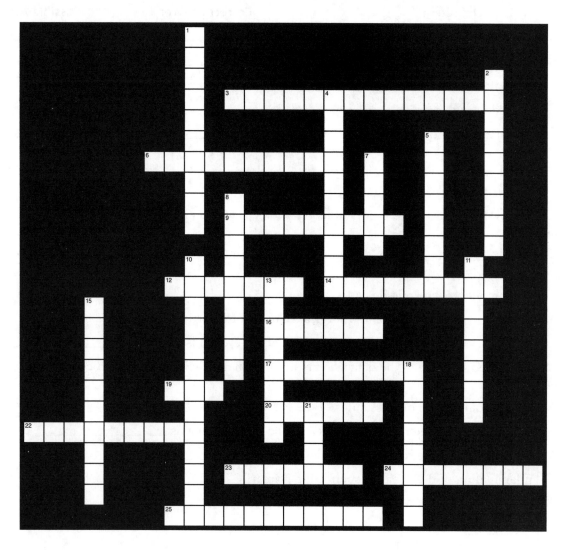

ACROSS

3. Also known as funduscopy
6. A fungal infection of the external auditory canal
9. Also known as cross-eyes
12. A sense of whirling, dizziness, and the loss of balance
14. An error of refraction
16. Accessory structures of an organ
17. The loss of transparency of the lens of the eye
19. Combining form meaning ear
20. Also known as nearsightedness
22. Common changes in the eye from aging
23. Combining form meaning eardrum
24. Discharge from the ear
25. Also known as choked disk

DOWN

1. Blindness in one half of the visual field
2. Also known as farsightedness
4. A condition in which the pupils are unequal in size
5. Combining form meaning eyelid
7. Suffix meaning hearing
8. Inflammation of the cornea
10. Also known as dry eye
11. Also known as double vision
13. Diseases characterized by increased intraocular pressure
15. A disorder in which the eyes point in different directions
18. A ringing, buzzing, or roaring sound in the ears
21. Suffix meaning vision condition

Skin: The Integumentary System

Learning Exercises

Class _____   Name _____

Matching Word Parts #1

Write the correct answer in the middle column.

Definition	Correct Answer	Possible Answers
12.1. dry	_____	cutane/o
12.2. skin	_____	rhytid/o
12.3. rash	_____	seb/o
12.4. sebum	_____	urtic/o
12.5. wrinkle	_____	xer/o

Matching Word Parts #2

Write the correct answer in the middle column.

Definition	Correct Answer	Possible Answers
12.6. black, dark	_____	kerat/o
12.7. fat, lipid	_____	lip/o
12.8. fungus	_____	melan/o
12.9. horny, hard	_____	myc/o
12.10. nail	_____	onych/o

Matching Word Parts #3

Write the correct answer in the middle column.

Definition	Correct Answer	Possible Answers
12.11. hairy	_____	dermat/o
12.12. hair	_____	hidr/o
12.13. pus	_____	hirsut/o
12.14. skin	_____	pil/i
12.15. sweat	_____	py/o

Fill in the Blank #1

12.16. A/An _____ is a cluster of connected boils.

12.17. A large blister, usually *more than* 0.5 cm in diameter, is known as a/an _____.

12.18. The highly contagious bacterial skin infection occurring in children and characterized by isolated pustules that become crusted and rupture is known as _____.

12.19. A/An _____ is a normal scar resulting from the healing of a wound.

12.20. A small, raised red lesion that is *less than* 0.5 cm in diameter and does not contain pus is known as a/an _____.

Word Construction #1

Use these word parts to construct the term that answers the following questions. Combining vowels are used in the term only when necessary. The answer includes the term (plus the appropriate word parts). For example: *hepatitis* (hepat, -itis).

-a	-derma	dermat/o	ecchym/o	-edema	erythem/o	hemat/o	-itis
lip/o	-oma	-osis	prurit/o	-rrhea	scler/o	seb/o	-us

12.21. A/An _____ is commonly known as a bruise.

12.22. Overactivity of the sebaceous glands that results in the production of an excessive amount of sebum is known as _____.

12.23. A/An _____ is a swelling of clotted blood trapped in the tissues.

12.24. A benign, slow-growing, fatty tumor located between the skin and the muscle layer is known as a/an _____.

12.25. The term _____ is used to describe an inflammation of the skin.

12.26. Redness of the skin due to capillary dilation is known as _____.

12.27. The condition known as _____ is an autoimmune disorder in which the connective tissues become thickened and hardened.

12.28. The condition characterized by the accumulation of fat and fluid in the tissues just under the skin of the hips and legs is known as _____.

12.29. The term _____ describes abnormal redness of the entire skin surface.

12.30. Commonly known as itching, the medical term for this condition is _____.

Matching Medical Terms and Definitions #1

Write the correct answer in the middle column.

Definitions	Correct Answer	Possible Answers
12.31. discolorations due to bleeding under the skin	_____	pediculosis
12.32. infestation with lice	_____	petechiae
12.33. pinpoint hemorrhages	_____	psoriasis
12.34. producing or containing pus	_____	purpura
12.35. red papules covered with silvery scales	_____	purulent

Word Surgery

Divide these terms into word parts, in the proper sequence, on the lines provided to create the answer to the question. Use a slash (/) to indicate a combining form. Use a hyphen to indicate a prefix or suffix. (You may not need all of the lines provided.)

12.36. The term **diaphoresis** means profuse sweating.

_____ _____ _____ _____

12.37. An inflammation of the hair follicles is known as **folliculitis**.

_____ _____ _____ _____

12.38. **Ichthyosis** is a group of hereditary disorders characterized by dry, thickened, and scaly skin.

_____ _____ _____ _____

12.39. Excessively dry skin is known as **xeroderma**.

_____ _____ _____ _____

12.40. **Koilonychia** is a malformation of the nails in which the outer surface is concave or scooped out like the bowl of a spoon.

_____ _____ _____ _____

Fill in the Blank #2

12.41. A/An _____ is a precancerous skin growth that occurs on sun-damaged skin. It often looks like a red, scaly patch and feels like sandpaper.

12.42. The medical term describing the autoimmune disorder characterized by a red, scaly rash on the face and upper trunk is systemic _____ (SLE).

12.43. The medical term _____ describes the condition in which there is widespread scaling of the skin, often with pruritus, erythroderma, and hair loss.

12.44. A/An _____ carcinoma originates as a malignant tumor of the scaly squamous cells of the epithelium; however, it can quickly spread to other body systems.

12.45. A/An _____ is a soft, raised, dark reddish-purple birthmark.

Multiple Choice

Select the correct answer and write it on the line provided.

12.46. The medical term for the condition commonly known as an ingrown toenail is _____.

onychocryptosis   onychomycosis

12.47. The skin condition resulting from the destruction of the melanocytes due to unknown causes is known as _____.

albinism   vitiligo

12.48. A/An _____ is a benign, superficial wartlike growth on the epithelial tissue.

papilloma   paronychia

12.49. A skin infection caused by an infestation with the itch mite is known as _____.

rosacea   scabies

12.50. A _____ is commonly known as a facelift.

blepharoplasty   rhytidectomy

Word Construction #2

Use these word parts to construct the term that answers the following questions. Combining vowels are used in the term only when necessary. The answer includes the term (plus the appropriate word parts). For example: *hepatitis* (hepat, -itis).

albin/o	alopec/o	-aria	blephar/o	-derma	dermat/o	granul/o
hirsut/o	-ia	-ism	-itis	kerat/o	melan/o	myc/o
-oma	onych/o	-osis	par-	-plasty	xer/o	

12.51. The term _____ describes a genetic condition characterized by a deficiency or the absence of pigment in the skin, hair, and irises of the eyes.

12.52. The term _____ means excessively dry skin.

12.53. The term _____ describes a fungal infection of the nail.

12.54. An acute or chronic infection of the skin fold around a nail is known as _____.

12.55. The term _____ describes the partial or complete loss of hair, most commonly on the scalp.

12.56. The term _____ describes any skin growth, such as a wart or a callus, in which there is overgrowth and thickening of the skin.

12.57. Malignant _____ is a type of skin cancer that occurs in the melanocytes.

12.58. A/An _____ is the surgical reduction of the upper and lower eyelids by removing excess fat, skin, and muscle.

12.59. The presence of excessive body and facial hair in women, usually occurring in a male pattern, is known as _____.

12.60. The general term used to describe small, knotlike swellings of granulation tissue in the epidermis is a/an _____.

Matching Medical Terms and Definitions #2

Write the correct answer in the middle column.

Definitions	Correct Answer	Possible Answers
12.61. abnormally thickened scar	_____	exanthem
12.62. also known as ringworm	_____	keloid
12.63. also known as warts	_____	tinea
12.64. widespread rash in children	_____	verrucae
12.65. small itchy bump	_____	wheal

Fill in the Blank #3

12.66. The chronic condition of unknown cause that produces redness, tiny pimples, and broken blood vessels is known as _____.

12.67. The term _____ describes an acute, rapidly spreading infection within the connective tissues.

12.68. The removal of dirt and debris from a wound to prevent infection and to promote healing is known as _____.

12.69. The severe infection caused by the pathogen known as flesh-eating bacteria is known as _____.

12.70. The condition known as _____, or the mask of pregnancy, is a pigmentation disorder characterized by brownish spots on the face.

12.71. A/An _____ is a noninfected lesion formed by the buildup of sebum and keratin in a hair follicle.

12.72. The condition known as _____ is a form of persistent or recurring dermatitis that is usually characterized by redness, itching, and dryness.

12.73. Atypical moles that can develop into skin cancer are known as _____.

12.74. A/An _____ is a small, flat, discolored spot such as a freckle.

12.75. A large, tender, swollen area caused by a staphylococcal infection around a hair follicle or sebaceous gland is known as a/an _____.

CHAPTER 12 CROSSWORD PUZZLE

The answers for this puzzle are located at the back of this workbook on page 104.

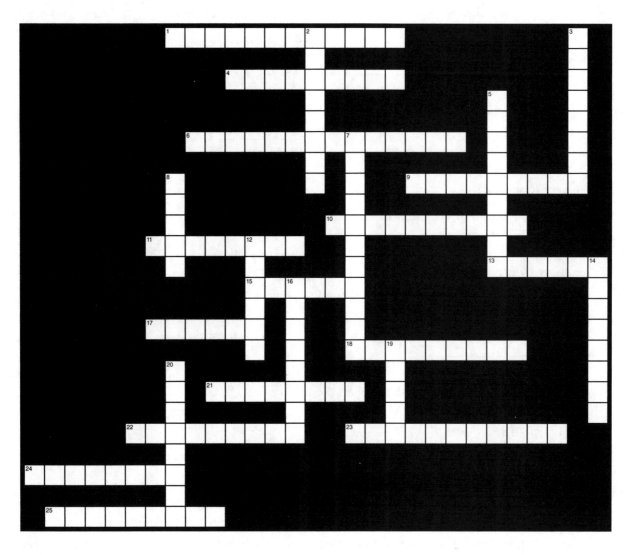

ACROSS

1. Also known as facelift
4. Also known as hives
6. Surgical reduction of the eyelids
9. Small knot-like swellings of granulation tissue
10. Also known as a bruise
11. Also known as warts
13. A small freckle or flat mole
15. Combining form meaning black
17. An abnormally raised or thickened scar
18. Overproduction of sebum
21. Also known as baldness
22. Excessively dry skin
23. Profuse sweating
24. Pus-producing
25. Overgrowth and thickening of the skin

DOWN

2. Normal scar
3. Redness of the skin due to capillary dilation
5. Excessive body and facial hair in women
7. Infestation with lice
8. Also known as ringworm
12. Non-infected lesion associated with acne vulgaris
14. Widespread rash, usually in children
16. A chronic abnormal accumulation of fat and fluid under the skin
19. Large blister
20. Also known as itching

The Endocrine System

Learning Exercises

Class _____   Name _____

Matching Word Parts #1

Write the correct answer in the middle column.

Definition	Correct Answer	Possible Answers
13.1. adrenal glands	_____	acr/o
13.2. extremities	_____	adren/o
13.3. sugar	_____	crin/o
13.4. thirst	_____	-dipsia
13.5. to secrete	_____	glyc/o

Matching Word Parts #2

Write the correct answer in the middle column.

Definition	Correct Answer	Possible Answers
13.6. condition	_____	gonad/o
13.7. sex glands	_____	-ism
13.8. pancreas	_____	pancreat/o
13.9. parathyroid glands	_____	parathyroid/o
13.10. pineal gland	_____	pineal/o

Matching Word Parts #3

Write the correct answer in the middle column.

Definition	Correct Answer	Possible Answers
13.11. body	_____	pituitar/o
13.12. many	_____	poly-
13.13. pituitary gland	_____	somat/o
13.14. thymus gland, soul	_____	thym/o
13.15. thyroid gland	_____	thyroid/o

Fill in the Blank #1

13.16. _____ disease occurs when the adrenal glands do not produce enough of the hormones cortisol or aldosterone.

13.17. _____ syndrome is caused by prolonged exposure to high levels of cortisol.

13.18. Mineral substances, such as sodium and potassium, that are normally found in the blood are known as _____.

13.19. The hormone _____ , which is secreted by the adrenal cortex, has an anti-inflammatory action. It also regulates the metabolism of carbohydrates, fats, and proteins in the body.

13.20. The hormone _____ is secreted by the thymus and stimulates the maturation of lymphocytes into T cells.

Word Construction #1

Use these word parts to construct the term that answers the following questions. Combining vowels are used in the term only when necessary. The answer includes the term (plus the appropriate word parts). For example: *hepatitis* (hepat, -itis).

acr/o	adrenal/o	-dipsia	-ectomy	insulin/o	-itis	lactin	-megaly
-oma	pancreat/o	-phagia	pineal/o	poly-	pro-	thym/o	-uria

13.21. An inflammation of the thymus gland is known as _____.

13.22. The term _____ describes abnormal enlargement of the extremities caused by the excessive secretion of growth hormone after puberty.

13.23. A benign tumor of the pancreas that causes hypoglycemia is known as _____.

13.24. The term _____ means excessive urination.

13.25. The surgical removal of the thymus gland is known as _____.

13.26. The term meaning excessive hunger is _____.

13.27. The medical term _____ describes inflammation of the adrenal glands.

13.28. A/An _____ is a benign tumor of the pituitary gland that causes excess production of prolactin.

13.29. An inflammation of the pancreas is known as _____.

13.30. The term _____ describes excessive thirst.

Matching Medical Terms and Definitions #1

Write the correct answer in the middle column.

Definitions	Correct Answer	Possible Answers
13.31. also known as blood sugar	_____	estrogen
13.32. develops female secondary sex characteristics	_____	glucagon
13.33. develops male secondary sex characteristics	_____	glucose
13.34. makes preparations for pregnancy	_____	progesterone
13.35. stimulates the liver to convert glycogen	_____	testosterone

Word Surgery

Divide these terms into word parts, in the proper sequence, on the lines provided to create the answer to the question. Use a slash (/) to indicate a combining form. Use a hyphen to indicate a prefix or suffix. (You may not need all of the lines provided.)

13.36. A **parathyroidectomy** is the surgical removal of one or more of the parathyroid glands.

_____ _____ _____ _____

13.37. The condition of excessive mammary development in the male is known as **gynecomastia**.

_____ _____ _____ _____

13.38. The condition of excessive secretion of insulin in the bloodstream is known as **hyperinsulinism**.

_____ _____ _____ _____

13.39. **Hypoglycemia** is an abnormally low concentration of glucose in the blood.

_____ _____ _____ _____

13.40. A benign tumor of the pancreas that causes hypoglycemia by secreting additional insulin is known as an **insulinoma**.

_____ _____ _____ _____

Fill in the Blank #2

13.41. The _____ hormone (ICSH) stimulates ovulation in the female. In the male, it stimulates the secretion of testosterone.

13.42. A minimally invasive procedure to surgically remove one or both adrenal glands is known as a/an _____.

13.43. The _____ hormone (FSH) stimulates the secretion of estrogen and the growth of ova in the female. In the male, it stimulates the production of sperm.

13.44. The _____ test measures average glucose levels over the past 3 weeks.

13.45. _____ syndrome is a disorder of the adrenal glands due to excessive production of aldosterone.

Multiple Choice

Select the correct answer and write it on the line provided.

13.46. The two primary thyroid hormones are _____ and triiodothyronine.

    thymosin   thyroxine

13.47. The hormone secreted by adipocytes (fat cells) is _____.

    leptin   oxytocin

13.48. The hormone _____ works with the parathyroid hormone to regulate the calcium levels in the blood and tissues.

    calcitonin   glycogen

13.49. The _____ hormone maintains the water balance within the body by promoting the reabsorption of water through the kidneys.

    antidiuretic   diuretic

13.50. The condition known as _____ is caused by insufficient production of the anti-diuretic hormone or by the inability of the kidneys to respond to this hormone.

    diabetes insipidus   diabetes mellitus

Word Construction #2

Use these word parts to construct the term that answers the following questions. Combining vowels are used in the term only when necessary. The answer includes the term (plus the appropriate word parts). For example: *hepatitis* (hepat, -itis).

calc/o	crin/o	-ectomy	-emia	glyc/o	hyper-
hypo-	-ia	-ism	parathyroid/o	pituitar/o	thyroid/o

13.51. The condition known as _____ is characterized by abnormally high concentrations of calcium circulating in the blood instead of being stored in the bones.

13.52. The term _____ describes the surgical removal of the parathyroid glands.

13.53. The condition known as _____ is caused by a deficiency of thyroid secretion.

13.54. An abnormally high concentration of glucose in the blood is known as _____.

13.55. The term _____ describes the excess secretion of growth hormone that causes acromegaly and gigantism.

Matching Medical Terms and Definitions #2

Write the correct answer in the middle column.

Definitions	Correct Answer	Possible Answers
13.56. abnormal overgrowth of body	_____	cretinism
13.57. congenital hypothyroidism	_____	gigantism
13.58. hormone-like substances	_____	myxedema
13.59. extreme thyroid deficiency	_____	puberty
13.60. change from child to adult	_____	steroids

Matching Medical Terms and Definitions #3

Write the correct answer in the middle column.

Definitions	Correct Answer	Possible Answers
13.61. abnormal protrusion of the eyeball	_____	prolactinoma
13.62. benign tumor of the pituitary gland	_____	oxytocin
13.63. occurs during some pregnancies	_____	norepinephrine
13.64. plays role in the fight-or-flight response	_____	gestational diabetes mellitus
13.65. stimulates contractions during childbirth	_____	exophthalmos

Fill in the Blank #3

13.66. The heart beats faster and blood pressure increases in response to _____, which is also known as adrenaline.

13.67. A/An _____ is a slow-growing, benign tumor of the pituitary gland.

13.68. The group of metabolic disorders characterized by hyperglycemia resulting from defects in insulin secretion, insulin action, or both is known as _____.

13.69. The _____ (LH) stimulates ovulation in the female and production of the female sex hormone progesterone.

13.70. The condition known as _____ is an abnormality of electrolyte balance caused by the excessive secretion of aldosterone.

13.71. An imbalance of metabolism caused by the overproduction of thyroid hormones is known as _____.

13.72. The oral administration of radioactive iodine to destroy thyroid cells is known as _____. (RAI).

13.73. The disorder known as _____ disease is an autoimmune disorder caused by hyperthyroidism that can also cause goiter and/or exophthalmos.

13.74. The autoimmune disorder in which the immune system mistakenly attacks thyroid tissue is known as _____.

13.75. Diabetic _____ occurs when diabetes damages the tiny blood vessels in the retina, causing blood to leak into the posterior segment of the eyeball.

CHAPTER 13 CROSSWORD PUZZLE

The answers for this puzzle are located at the back of this workbook on page 105.

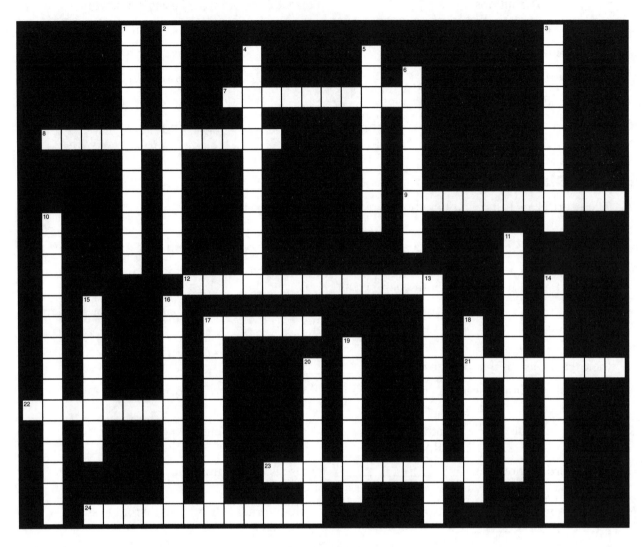

ACROSS

7. Excessive hunger
8. Mineral substances normally found in the blood
9. Inflammation of the adrenal glands
12. Abnormally high concentration of glucose in the blood
17. Combining form meaning adrenal
21. Hormone important in the regulation of the menstrual cycle
22. The hormone secreted by the pancreatic islets in response to low blood sugar levels
23. Blood sugar level is higher than normal
24. Abnormally low concentration of glucose in the blood

DOWN

1. Abnormal protrusion of the eyes
2. Excessive mammary development in the male
3. Excessive thirst
4. Hormone released during the second half of the menstrual cycle
5. Abnormal growth of the body prior to puberty
6. Combining form meaning pancreas
10. Excessive secretion of insulin that can cause hypoglycemia
11. A benign tumor of the pituitary gland
13. Hormone that regulates salt and water levels within the body
14. Hormone that stimulates the development of male secondary sex characteristics
15. Hormone that stimulates uterine contractions
16. Hormone that stimulates ovulation
17. Hormonal disorder causing enlarged extremities
18. A congenital form of hypothyroidism
19. Inflammation of the thymus gland
20. A severe form of adult hypothyroidism

The Reproductive Systems

Learning Exercises

Class _____   Name _____

Matching Word Parts #1

Write the correct answer in the middle column.

Definition	Correct Answer	Possible Answers
14.1. cervix	_____	cervic/o
14.2. female	_____	colp/o
14.3. pregnant	_____	-gravida
14.4. uterus	_____	gynec/o
14.5. vagina	_____	hyster/o

Matching Word Parts #2

Write the correct answer in the middle column.

Definition	Correct Answer	Possible Answers
14.6. breast	_____	mast/o
14.7. egg	_____	men/o
14.8. menstruation	_____	orchid/o
14.9. testicles	_____	ov/o
14.10. ovary	_____	ovari/o

Matching Word Parts #3

Write the correct answer in the middle column.

Definition	Correct Answer	Possible Answers
14.11. to bring forth	_____	-para
14.12. surgical fixation	_____	-pexy
14.13. tube	_____	salping/o
14.14. testicle	_____	test/i, test/o
14.15. vagina	_____	vagin/o

Fill in the Blank #1

14.16. The STD known as _____ is caused by the bacterium *Treponema pallidum* and is highly contagious.

14.17. A/An _____ pregnancy is a potentially dangerous condition in which a fertilized egg is implanted and begins to develop outside of the uterus.

14.18. The evaluation of a newborn infant's physical status at 1 and 5 minutes after birth is known as a/an _____ score.

14.19. A/An _____ sampling (CVS) is performed between the 8th and 10th weeks of pregnancy to search for genetic abnormalities in the developing fetus.

14.20. The condition known as _____ is characterized by convulsions and sometimes coma, and is treated by delivery of the fetus.

Word Construction #1

Use these word parts to construct the term that answers the following questions. Combining vowels are used in the term only when necessary. The answer includes the term (plus the appropriate word parts). For example: *hepatitis* (hepat, -itis).

cervic/o	colp/o	-ectomy	endo-	epididym/o	episi/o	-itis	metri/o
orchid/o	-osis	-otomy	ovari/o	-pexy	-rrhaphy	-rrhexis	-scopy

14.21. The term _____ describes rupture of an ovary.

14.22. A/An _____ is the surgical fixation of a prolapsed vagina to a surrounding structure such as the abdominal wall.

14.23. The endoscopic surgery to move an undescended testicle into its normal position in the scrotum is known as a/an _____.

14.24. A/An _____ is a surgical incision made to prevent tearing of the tissues as the infant moves out of the birth canal.

14.25. The condition known as _____ is an inflammation of the mucous membrane lining of the cervix.

14.26. The surgical suturing of a tear in the vagina is known as a/an _____.

14.27. A/An _____ is the surgical removal of one or both testicles.

14.28. The condition in which patches of endometrial tissue become attached to other structures in the pelvic cavity is known as _____.

14.29. The procedure known as _____ is the direct visual examination of the tissues of the cervix and vagina.

14.30. An inflammation of the epididymis is known as _____.

Matching Medical Terms and Definitions #1

Write the correct answer in the middle column.

Definitions	Correct Answer	Possible Answers
14.31. caused by *Chlamydia trachomatis*	_____	andropause
14.32. caused by *Neisseria gonorrhoeae*	_____	chlamydia
14.33. caused by *Trichomonas vaginalis*	_____	colostrum
14.34. male menopause	_____	gonorrhea
14.35. milk produced after giving birth	_____	trichomoniasis

Word Surgery

Divide these terms into word parts, in the proper sequence, on the lines provided to create the answer to the question. Use a slash (/) to indicate a combining form. Use a hyphen to indicate a prefix or suffix. (You may not need all of the lines provided.)

14.36. **Amniocentesis** is a surgical puncture with a needle to obtain a specimen of amniotic fluid.

_____ _____ _____ _____

14.37. **Perimenopause** is the term used to designate the transition phase between regular menstrual periods and no periods at all.

_____ _____ _____ _____

14.38. The term **galactorrhea** describes the production of breast milk in a woman who is not breastfeeding.

_____ _____ _____ _____

14.39. **Menometrorrhagia** is excessive uterine bleeding both at the usual time of menstrual periods and at other irregular intervals.

_____ _____ _____ _____

14.40. The term **menarche** describes the beginning of the menstrual function.

_____ _____ _____ _____

Fill in the Blank #2

14.41. _____ disease is a sexual dysfunction in which the penis is bent or curved during erection.

14.42. A/An _____ (SO) is the surgical removal of a fallopian tube and ovary.

14.43. The term _____ describes a condition of severe itching of the external female genitalia.

14.44. A/An _____ specializes in providing medical care to women during pregnancy and childbirth, and immediately thereafter.

14.45. A/An _____ is a round, firm, rubbery mass that arises from excess growth of glandular and connective tissue in the breast.

Multiple Choice

Select the correct answer and write it on the line provided.

14.46. The term _____ describes the absence of sperm in the semen.

    azoospermia   hematospermia

14.47. The term _____ describes a woman who has never borne a viable child.

    nulligravida   nullipara

14.48. Mammoplasty that is performed to affix sagging breasts in a more elevated position is known as _____.

    mastalgia   mastopexy

14.49. The term used to describe infrequent or very light menstruation in a woman with previously normal periods is _____.

    hypomenorrhea   oligomenorrhea

14.50. A _____ is a woman during her first pregnancy.

    primigravida   primipara

Word Construction #2

Use these word parts to construct the term that answers the following questions. Combining vowels are used in the term only when necessary. The answer includes the term (plus the appropriate word parts). For example: *hepatitis* (hepat, -itis).

a-	-algia	-cele	cervic/o	dys-	-ectomy
hemat/o	hydr/o	hypo-	hyster/o	-ia	-itis
leuk/o	mast/o	men/o	metr/o	-rrhea	sperm/o

14.51. The term _____ describes an abnormal discharge, such as mucus or pus, from the uterus.

14.52. An inflammation of the cervix that is usually caused by an infection is known as _____.

14.53. A/An _____ is a fluid-filled sac in the scrotum along the spermatic cord leading from the testicles.

14.54. An abnormal absence of menstrual periods for 90 or more days is known as _____.

14.55. The term _____ means pain in the breast.

14.56. The term _____ describes a profuse whitish mucus discharge from the uterus and vagina.

14.57. Pain caused by uterine cramps during a menstrual period is known as _____.

14.58. The term _____ describes the presence of blood in the seminal fluid.

14.59. A/An _____ is the surgical removal of the uterus.

14.60. An usually small amount of menstrual flow during a shortened regular menstrual period is known as _____.

Matching Medical Terms and Definitions #2

Write the correct answer in the middle column.

Definitions	Correct Answer	Possible Answers
14.61. benign cysts in the breasts	_____	cervical dysplasia
14.62. first 4 weeks of life	_____	fibrocystic breast disease
14.63. has borne one viable child	_____	neonate
14.64. never been pregnant	_____	nulligravida
14.65. precancerous lesions	_____	primipara

Fill in the Blank #3

14.66. The diagnostic procedure known as _____(HSG) is a specialized radiographic examination of the uterus and fallopian tubes.

14.67. A/An _____ is a procedure performed as an attempt to restore fertility to a vasectomized male.

14.68. The abnormal implantation of the placenta in the lower portion of the uterus is known as _____.

14.69. In the _____ syndrome, the ovaries are enlarged by the presence of many cysts formed by incompletely developed follicles.

14.70. A/An _____ is the condition in which the uterus slides from its normal position and sags into the vagina.

14.71. The direct visual examination of the interior of the uterus and fallopian tubes is known as _____.

14.72. The term _____ describes a complication of pregnancy that is also known as pregnancy-induced hypertension.

14.73. A/An _____ is a knot of varicose veins in one side of the scrotum.

14.74. The surgical removal of one or both ovaries is known as a/an _____.

14.75. A/An _____ is a painful erection that lasts 4 hours or more.

CHAPTER 14 CROSSWORD PUZZLE

The answers for this puzzle are located at the back of this workbook on page 106.

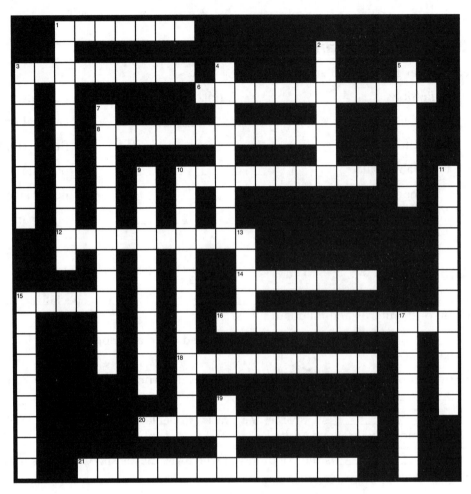

ACROSS

1. Combining form meaning uterus
3. Surgical fixation of sagging breasts in a more elevated position
6. Pain caused by uterine cramps during a menstrual period
8. A Woman who has never been pregnant
10. Surgery to move an undescended testicle into its normal position
12. An abnormal discharge from the uterus
14. Suffix meaning pregnant
15. Combining form meaning vagina
16. Also known as pregnancy-induced hypertension
18. A surgical incision through the perineum to prevent the tearing of tissue during childbirth
20. Specialist in care of women during pregnancy
21. An STD also known as trich

DOWN

1. Surgical removal of the uterus
2. A newborn infant
3. The beginning of the menstrual function
4. A fluid-filled sac in the scrotum
5. Combining form meaning cervix
7. A condition in which endometrial tissue escapes the uterus
9. The absense of sperm in the semen
10. The rupture of an ovary
11. A woman during her first pregnancy
13. Score to evaluate a newborn infant's physical status
15. Surgical fixation of a prolapsed vagina to a surrounding structure
17. Combining form meaning fallopian tube
19. Combining form meaning menstruation

Diagnostic Procedures, Nuclear Medicine, and Pharmacology

Learning Exercises

Class _____   Name _____

Matching Word Parts #1

Write the correct answer in the middle column.

Definition	Correct Answer	Possible Answers
15.1. albumin, protein	_____	albumin/o
15.2. calcium	_____	calc/i
15.3. creatinine	_____	-centesis
15.4. sugar	_____	creatin/o
15.5. surgical puncture for the removal of fluid	_____	glycos/o

Matching Word Parts #2

Write the correct answer in the middle column.

Definition	Correct Answer	Possible Answers
15.6. abdomen	_____	phleb/o
15.7. blood	_____	-otomy
15.8. process of producing a picture or record	_____	lapar/o
15.9. surgical incision	_____	hemat/o
15.10. vein	_____	-graphy

Matching Word Parts #3

Write the correct answer in the middle column.

Definition	Correct Answer	Possible Answers
15.11. direct visual examination	_____	radi/o
15.12. radiation	_____	-scope
15.13. sound	_____	-scopy
15.14. urine	_____	son/o
15.15. visual examination instrument	_____	-uria

Fill in the Blank #1

15.16. The patient's consistency and accuracy in following the regimen prescribed by a physician or other health care professional is referred to as _____.

15.17. A/An _____ is an abnormal sound heard during auscultation of an artery.

15.18. The term _____ means listening for sounds within the body and is usually performed through a stethoscope.

15.19. The medication that acts as an analgesic to reduce pain and fever but does not relieve inflammation is _____.

15.20. The term _____ describes any position in which the patient is lying down.

Word Construction #1

Use these word parts to construct the term that answers the following questions. Combining vowels are used in the term only when necessary. The answer includes the term (plus the appropriate word parts). For example: *hepatitis* (hepat, -itis).

albumin/o	an-	arthr/o	bacteri/o	calci/o	cardi/o	-centesis
glycos/o	hemat/o	keton/o	peri-	protein/o	py/o	-uria

15.21. The presence of pus in urine is known as _____.

15.22. The surgical puncture of the joint space to remove synovial fluid for analysis is known as _____.

15.23. The term _____ describes the presence of glucose in the urine.

15.24. A sign of impaired kidney function is the presence of the protein albumin in the urine. This condition is known as _____.

15.25. The term _____ describes the puncture of the pericardial sac for the purpose of removing fluid.

15.26. The presence of an abnormal amount of protein in the urine is known as _____.

15.27. The term _____ describes presence of blood in the urine.

15.28. The presence of calcium in the urine is known as _____.

15.29. The term _____ describes the presence of ketones in the urine. Their presence in urine can indicate starvation or uncontrolled diabetes.

15.30. The presence of bacteria in urine is known as _____.

Matching Examination Instruments and Definitions

Write the correct answer in the middle column.

Definitions	Correct Answer	Possible Answers
15.31. enlarge opening of body canal	_____	ophthalmoscope
15.32. examine external ear canal	_____	otoscope
15.33. examine interior of eye	_____	speculum
15.34. listen to sounds within body	_____	sphygmomanometer
15.35. measures blood pressure	_____	stethoscope

Word Surgery

Divide these terms into word parts, in the proper sequence, on the lines provided to create the answer to the question. Use a slash (/) to indicate a combining form. Use a hyphen to indicate a prefix or suffix. (You may not need all of the lines provided.)

15.36. **Phlebotomy** is the puncture of a vein for the purpose of drawing blood.

_____   _____   _____   _____

15.37. A medication administered to prevent or reduce fever is known as an **antipyretic**.

_____   _____   _____   _____

15.38. **Laparoscopy** is the visual examination of the interior of the abdomen with the use of a laparoscope that is passed through a small incision in the abdominal wall.

_____   _____   _____   _____

15.39. A **transdermal** medication is administered from a patch that is applied to unbroken skin.

_____   _____   _____   _____

15.40. Imaging of deep body structures by recording the echoes of pulses of sound waves that are above the range of human hearing is known as **ultrasonography**.

_____   _____   _____   _____

Fill in the Blank #2

15.41. The term _____ describes a substance that does not allow x-rays to pass through. These substances appear white or light gray on the resulting film.

15.42. The technique known as _____ (CT) uses a thin, fan-shaped x-ray beam that rotates around the patient to produce multiple cross-sectional views of the body.

15.43. A/An _____ is a factor in the patient's condition that makes the use of a medication or specific treatment dangerous or ill advised.

15.44. The term _____ describes the flow of blood through an organ.

15.45. The technique known as _____ (MRI) uses a combination of radio waves and a strong magnetic field to create images of any body plane.

Multiple Choice

Select the correct answer and write it on the line provided.

15.46. The term _____ means that the substance allows x-rays to pass through and appears black or dark gray on the resulting film.

    radiolucent   radiopaque

15.47. An abnormally low body temperature is known as _____.

    hyperthermia   hypothermia

15.48. A _____ is a substance that eases the pain or severity of the symptoms of a disease but does not cure it.

    palliative   placebo

15.49. Coarse rattling sounds caused by secretions in the bronchial airways are known as _____.

    rhonchi   stridor

15.50. The diagnostic procedure known as _____ is designed to determine the density of a body part by the sound produced by tapping the surface with the fingers.

    parenteral   percussion

Word Construction #2

Use these word parts to construct the term that answers the following questions. Combining vowels are used in the term only when necessary. The answer includes the term (plus the appropriate word parts). For example: *hepatitis* (hepat, -itis).

        cardi/o   creatin/o   -crit   echo-   fluor/o   -graphy

        hemat/o   hyper-   -ia   -scopy   therm/o   -uria

15.51. The visualization of body parts in motion by projecting x-ray images on a luminous fluorescent screen is known as _____.

15.52. The term _____ describes an increased concentration of creatinine in the urine.

15.53. _____ describes the percentage, by volume, of a blood sample occupied by red cells.

15.54. The ultrasonic diagnostic procedure used to evaluate the structures and motion of the heart is known as _____.

15.55. The term _____ describes an extremely high fever.

Fill in the Blank #3

15.56. Single _____ computed tomography (**SPECT**) is a type of nuclear imaging test that produces 3-D computer-reconstructed images.

15.57. A/An _____ is an unexpected reaction to a drug that is peculiar to the individual.

15.58. Positron _____ (**PET**) combines tomography with radionuclide tracers to produce enhanced images of selected body organs or areas.

15.59. The examination of the physical and chemical properties of urine to determine the presence of abnormal elements is known as _____.

15.60. An ultrasonic imaging technique used to evaluate heart structures is known as _____(TEE).

Matching Medical Terms and Definitions

Write the correct answer in the middle column.

Definitions	Correct Answer	Possible Answers
15.61. administered for suggestive effects	_____	acupuncture
15.62. cracklelike respiratory sound	_____	parenteral
15.63. high-pitched, abnormal harsh sound	_____	placebo
15.64. Chinese medical practice using needles	_____	rale
15.65. not administered through the digestive tract	_____	stridor

Fill in the Blank #4

15.66. A/An _____ injection (SC) is made into the fatty layer just below the skin.

15.67. A diagnostic instrument that is a small, flexible tube with a light and a lens on the end is known as a/an _____.

15.68. In the _____ position, the patient is lying on the left side with the right knee and thigh drawn up with the left arm placed along the back.

15.69. The term _____ refers to the class of drugs that relieves pain without affecting consciousness.

15.70. A/An _____ injection is made into the middle layers of the skin.

15.71. The use of radiographic imaging to guide a procedure is known as _____.

15.72. In a _____ position, the patient is lying on the abdomen with the face down.

15.73. The type of injection made directly into muscle tissue is known as a/an _____ (IM).

15.74. In the _____ position, the patient is lying on the back with the feet and legs raised and supported in stirrups. This position is used for vaginal and rectal examinations.

15.75. A/An _____ injection (IV) is made directly into a vein.

CHAPTER 15 CROSSWORD PUZZLE

The answers for this puzzle are located at the back of this workbook on page 107.

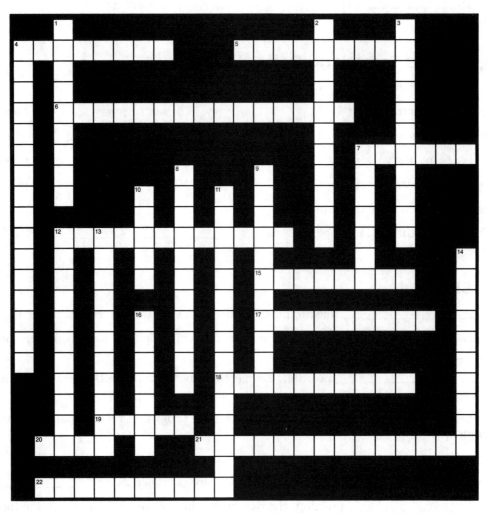

ACROSS

4. Instrument used to enlarge a body opening
5. The presence of ketones in the urine
6. Echocardiography performed from inside the esophagus
7. Pus in the urine
12. Listening through a stethoscope
15. Instrument to examine the external ear canal
17. The presence of calcium in the urine
18. The presence of glucose in the urine
19. Position with patient lying on the abdomen, face down
20. Abnormal rattle or crackle-like respiratory sound
21. Instrument used to examine the interior of the eye
22. Puncture of a vein for the purpose of drawing blood

DOWN

1. The presence of blood in the urine
2. Injection into the middle layers of the skin
3. Allows x-rays to pass through
4. Instrument used to measure blood pressure
7. A substance given for its suggestive effects
8. The presence of bacteria in the urine
9. Projecting x-ray images of body parts in motion on a fluorescent screen
10. Abnormal sound or murmur heard in auscultation
11. The use of sound waves to image deep body structure
12. The presence of albumin in the urine
13. Instrument used to listen to sounds within the body
14. Does not allow x-rays to pass through
16. An abnormal, high-pitched, harsh sound heard during inhalation

Answers to Crossword Puzzles

CHAPTER 1 CROSSWORD PUZZLE ANSWER KEY

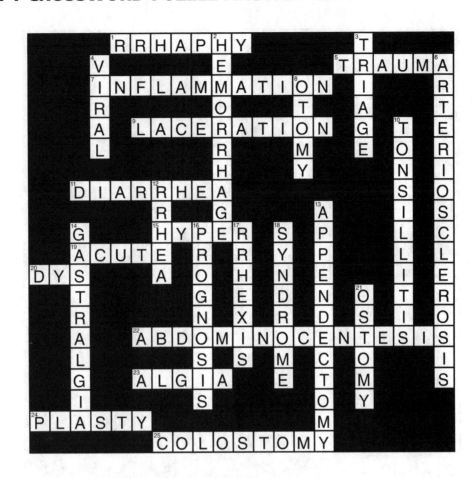

CHAPTER 2 CROSSWORD PUZZLE ANSWER KEY

```
            A D E N E C T O M Y        A
      A       N                        D
      N O S O C O M I A L        I     E
      T       M         D      H O     N
      C E P H A L I C   I      O N     O
      R       L     E   C O N G E N I T A L
      I       Y   E N   Y     O N       L
      O           N D   T   D I S T A L
              E T I O L O G Y   T     L
    E         X   D     P   S   A
    P A T H O     I     L   P O S T E R I O R
    I           O     A   L       I
    G             P L A S I A S   S
    A P L A S I A     M   S
    S           T     H I S T O L O G Y
    T           H         A
    R     P R O X I M A L
    I           C
    C A U D A L
```

Across: ADENECTOMY, NOSOCOMIAL, CEPHALIC, CONGENITAL, DISTAL, ETIOLOGY, PATHO, POSTERIOR, PLASIA, APLASIA, HISTOLOGY, PROXIMAL, CAUDAL

Down: ANOMALY, ADENOMA, ANTERIOR, DIP, HOMONY, INGUINAL, ENDO, CYTO, PLASIA, EPIGASTRIC, DIOA, IDIOPATHIC

CHAPTER 3 CROSSWORD PUZZLE ANSWER KEY

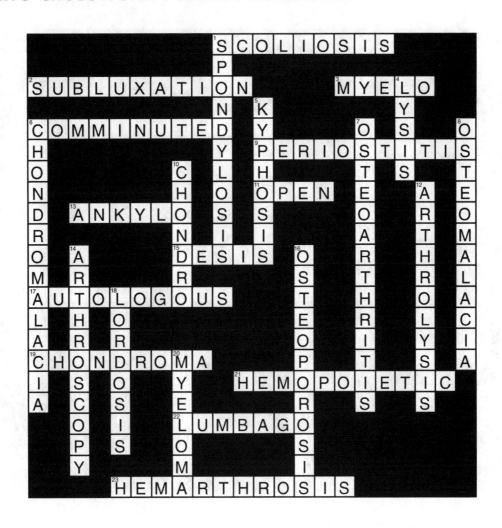

CHAPTER 4 CROSSWORD PUZZLE ANSWER KEY

CHAPTER 5 CROSSWORD PUZZLE ANSWER KEY

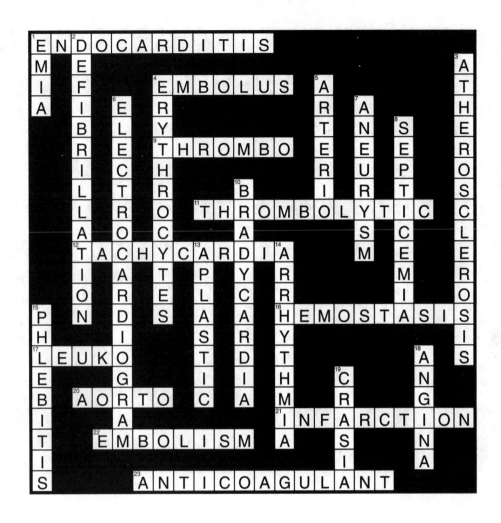

CHAPTER 6 CROSSWORD PUZZLE ANSWER KEY

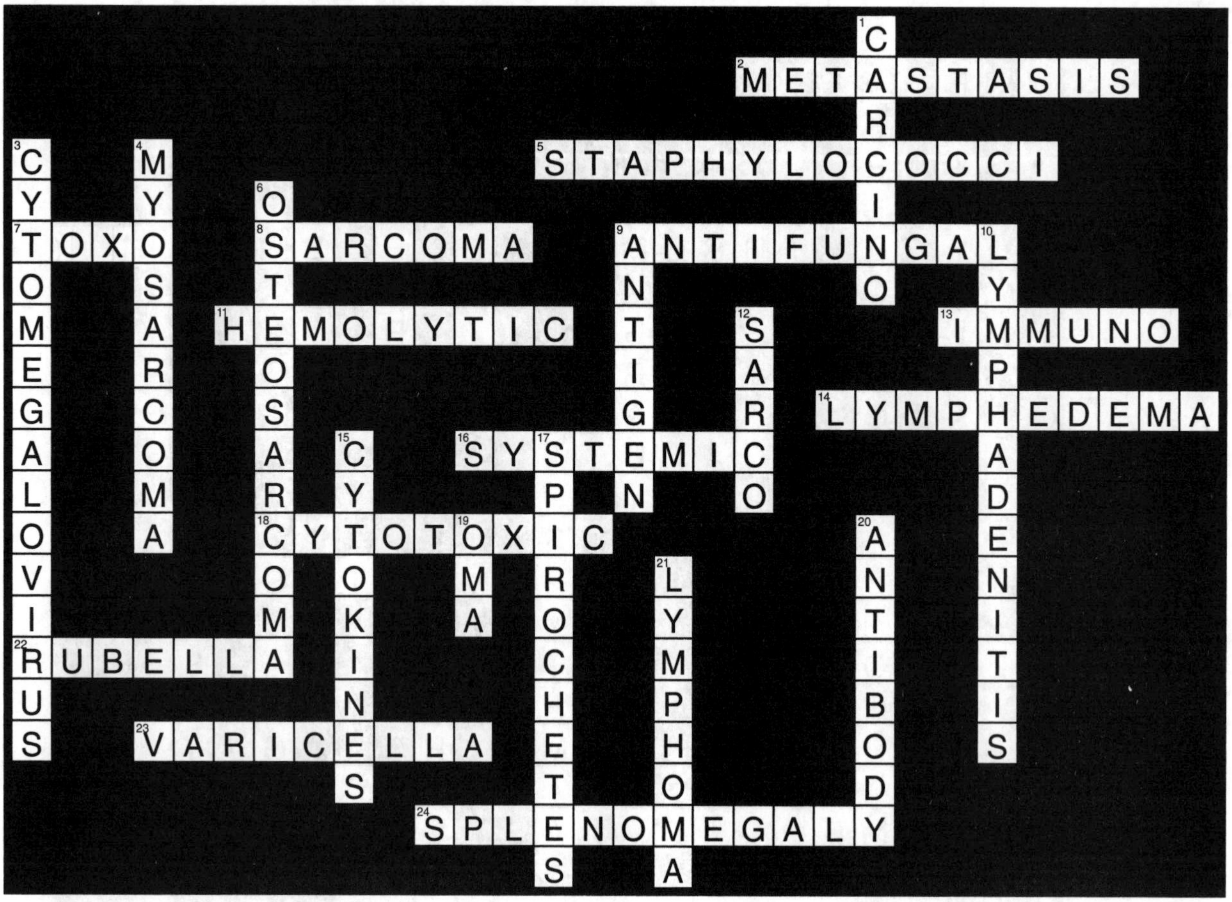
1 CARCINO
2 METASTASIS
3 CYTOMEGALOVIRUS
4 MYOSARCOMA
5 STAPHYLOCOCCI
6 OSTEOSARCOMA
7 TOXO
8 SARCOMA
9 ANTIFUNGAL
9 ANTIGEN
10 LYMPHADENITIS
11 HEMOLYTIC
12 SARCO
13 IMMUNO
14 LYMPHEDEMA
15 CYTOKINES
16 SYSTEMIC
17 SPIROCHETES
18 CYTOTOXIC
19 OMA
20 ANTIBODY
21 LYMPHOMA
22 RUBELLA
23 VARICELLA
24 SPLENOMEGALY

CHAPTER 7 CROSSWORD PUZZLE ANSWER KEY

CHAPTER 8 CROSSWORD PUZZLE ANSWER KEY

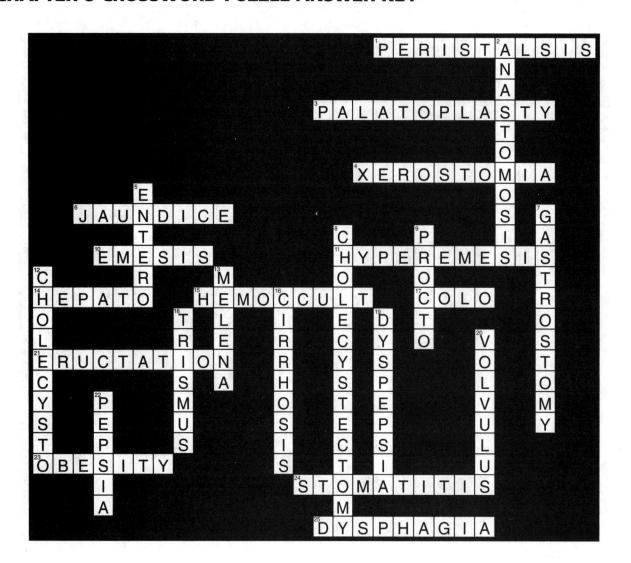

CHAPTER 9 CROSSWORD PUZZLE ANSWER KEY

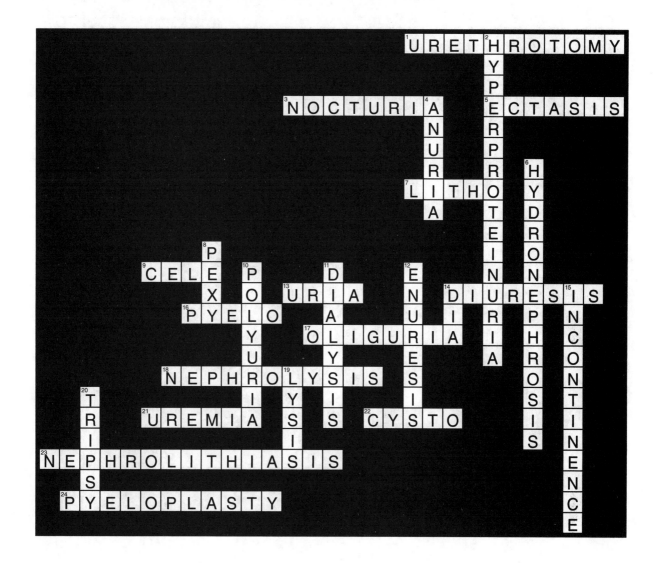

CHAPTER 10 CROSSWORD PUZZLE ANSWER KEY

```
                                    ¹C
                         ²D E L I R I U M              ⁵N
      ⁶H                   E    A    A    E             A
      A                    L    U    D    N             R
      L         ⁷E         U    S    I    I             C
      L         N          S    T    C    N             O
      U         C          I    R    U    G             L
      C         E        ⁸M Y E L O  O    I    ⁹M       E
      I         P          N    P    L    T    Y        P
      N         H          ¹⁰E P I L E P S Y            S
    ¹¹P A R E S T H E S I A  ¹²S Y N C O P E  S    L    Y
      A         A           B         B         I    ¹³H
      T         L  ¹⁴C O N ¹⁵C U S S I O N   ¹⁶L E T H A R G Y
      I         A        O   A               I    Y
      O    ¹⁷H E M O R R H A G I C           S    P
      N              N                            E
         ¹⁸E  ¹⁹D    I                            R
         S    Y   ²⁰S ²¹C I A T I C A             E
         T    S    O  O                           S
         H    L    M  M                           T
       ²²D E M E N T I A  ²³E N C E P H A L I T I S H
         S    X    I                              E
         I    I    O                              S
         A    A                  ²⁴S C H I Z O P H R E N I A
```

CHAPTER 11 CROSSWORD PUZZLE ANSWER KEY

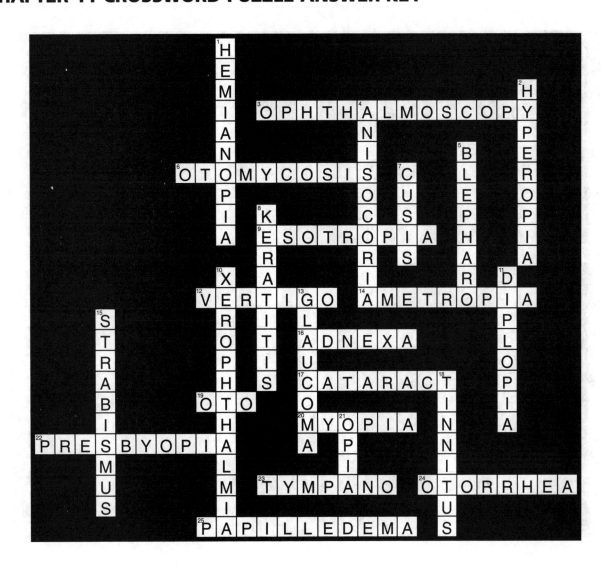

CHAPTER 12 CROSSWORD PUZZLE ANSWER KEY

```
1 R H Y T I D E C T O M Y                    3 E
        C                                      R
    4 U R T I C A R I A                        Y
        A                                      T
        T                          5 H         H
    6 B L E P H A R O P L A S T Y   I          E
        R             E             R          M
        I             D   9 G R A N U L O M A  A
    8 T I N E       10 E C C H Y M O S I S
      I X             D             T
  11 V E R R U C A E  U             I
    A     12 O        L             S  13 M A C U L E 14 E
          M 16 15 M E L A N O       S             X
          E   P     S                             A
  17 K E L O I D     I 18 19 S E B O R R H E A     N
          O   P       20 U                        T
        P R U L E C I A   L                        H
        R   I M 21 A L O P E C I A                 E
        U   T     D       L                        M
  22 X E R O D E R M A   23 D I A P H O R E S I S
        I   U
  24 P U R U L E N T
        U
  25 K E R A T O S I S
```

CHAPTER 13 CROSSWORD PUZZLE ANSWER KEY

CHAPTER 14 CROSSWORD PUZZLE ANSWER KEY

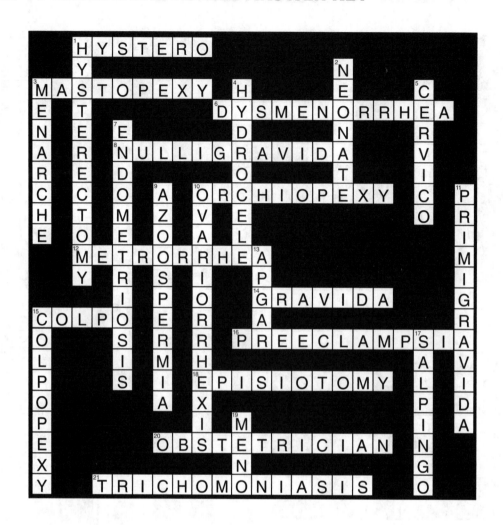

CHAPTER 15 CROSSWORD PUZZLE ANSWER KEY

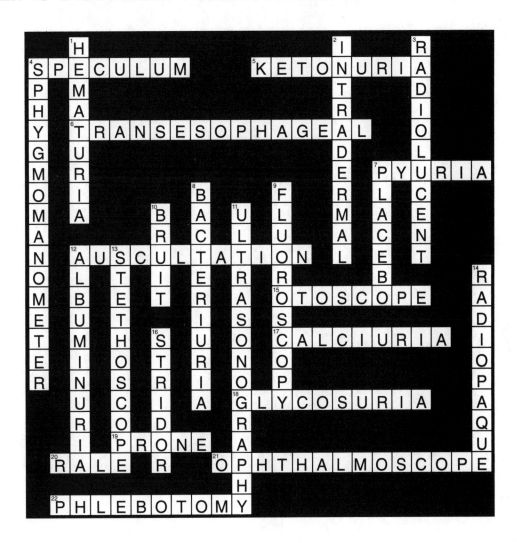